STUDENT UNIT

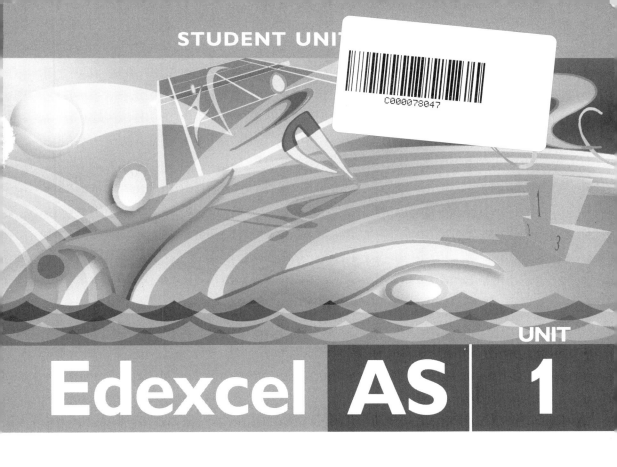

Edexcel AS

UNIT

1

Physical Education

Participation in Sport and Recreation

Mike Hill and Gavin Roberts

Philip Allan Updates, an imprint of Hodder Education, part of Hachette Livre UK, Market Place, Deddington, Oxfordshire OX15 0SE

Orders

Bookpoint Ltd, 130 Milton Park, Abingdon, Oxfordshire OX14 4SB
tel: 01235 827720
fax: 01235 400454
e-mail: uk.orders@bookpoint.co.uk
Lines are open 9.00 a.m.–5.00 p.m., Monday to Saturday, with a 24-hour message answering service. You can also order through the Philip Allan Updates website: www.philipallan.co.uk

© Philip Allan Updates 2008

ISBN 978-0-340-96676-1

First printed 2008
Impression number   5 4 3 2 1
Year   2013 2012 2011 2010 2009 2008

This guide has been written specifically to support students preparing for the Edexcel AS Physical Education Unit 1 examination. The content has been neither approved nor endorsed by Edexcel and remains the sole responsibility of the authors.

Typeset by Phoenix Photosetting, Chatham, Kent
Printed by MPG Books, Bodmin

Hachette Livre UK's policy is to use papers that are natural, renewable and recyclable products and made from wood grown in sustainable forests. The logging and manufacturing processes are expected to conform to the environmental regulations of the country of origin.

Contents

Introduction

■ ■ ■

Content Guidance

■ ■ ■

Questions and Answers

Introduction

About this guide

This guide is the first in a series of four that cover the whole Edexcel specification for AS and A-level physical education. Its aim is to help you prepare for the Unit 1 test by providing an understanding of the key concepts, as well as looking at revision strategies and examination techniques. It is divided into three sections:

- **Introduction** — this provides advice on how to use the guide, an explanation of the skills required in AS PE, and suggestions for effective revision. It also offers guidance on how to apply your knowledge in the examination.
- **Content Guidance** — this summarises the specification content of Unit 1.
- **Questions and Answers** — this contains mock questions for you to try, together with sample answers to the questions and examiner's comments on how these answers could be improved. Each question has been attempted by two candidates, Candidate A and Candidate B. Their answers, along with the examiner's comments, should help you to see what you need to do to achieve a good grade. They also demonstrate how you can easily miss marks even though you may understand the topic.

Content Guidance

The specification content is divided into two sections. The first section investigates what constitutes a healthy and active lifestyle; the second considers how competitive sport has developed over time.

Healthy and active lifestyles

The section begins with a review of the development of active leisure and recreation, and an examination of contemporary concerns to individuals and society about health and fitness. Key concepts include:

- the basic requirements for sport and leisure
- the concepts of recreation, active leisure, health, fitness and exercise
- the relationship between nutrition and weight management
- current trends in health and fitness
- the components of a balanced lifestyle
- the effects of ageing and their impact on access to sport and recreation
- the effects of exercise
- fitness and training

Opportunities and pathways

In this second part of the unit a sociological view of sport is discussed. This begins with a review of the way in which competitive sport in the UK has developed, and examines the effect that this development has had on current provision for both sport and recreation.

Key concepts include:

- the role of festivals in the historical development of sport in the UK
- the emergence of rational sport linked to the Industrial Revolution of the nineteenth century
- the further development of sport, particularly increasing commercialisation and globalisation

The unit then moves on to look at performance pathways in sport at both local and national levels (this links to the coursework tasks in Unit 2). This involves looking at elite sports pathways, for example how a performer moves from foundation level to playing at international level. It also looks at access into the performance pathway, and how and why some groups in society may find this more difficult.

In the final part of the unit there is an investigation into the current model of long-term athlete development. This model has been adopted by most national governing bodies for sport in the UK.

How should I use this guide?

The guide can be used throughout your physical education course — it is not *just* a revision aid. Because the Content Guidance is laid out in sections that correspond to those of the specification for Unit 1, you can use it:

- to check that your notes cover the material required by the specification
- to identify strengths and weaknesses
- as a reference for homework and internal tests
- during your revision to prepare 'bite-sized' chunks of related material, rather than being faced with a file full of notes

The Question and Answer section can be used to:

- identify the terms used by examiners in questions and what they expect of you
- familiarise yourself with the style of questions you can expect
- identify the ways in which marks are lost as well as the ways in which they are gained

The specification

To make a good start to studying Unit 1, you need to have access to the unit specification. This can be obtained from your teacher or directly from the awarding body, Edexcel, at **www.edexcel.org.uk**.

The specification identifies everything that needs to be covered and understood. It also informs you as to what could be in the end-of-unit examination — if a topic is in the specification, then it could be examined; if it is not, it will not be examined.

Study skills and revision strategies

Revision and preparation for examinations are very personal. However, there are common approaches that should be employed by all. Being successful in any subject depends on:

- understanding — the ability to follow a particular concept
- learning — the ability to recall the concept without prompts
- application — the ability to use the knowledge you have learnt to answer the questions that have been asked

The Question and Answer section of this guide deals with application.

Past papers can be very useful. They will familiarise you with the format of the questions and the language used. There are also mark schemes and examiners' reports available. These indicate the sorts of mistakes made by students when faced with particular questions. They also include some model answers.

There are several ways of learning and individuals will have particular favourites determined by their preferred learning style(s), whether it is auditory, visual or kinaesthetic. However, there are common areas of good practice that should be adopted by all students. Whatever your preferred style, you must work out a revision plan.

What you must do

- Leave yourself enough time to cover all the material identified in the Unit 1 specification.
- Make sure that you have all the material to hand (use this book as a basis).
- Identify weaknesses early in your preparation so that you have time to do something about them.
- Familiarise yourself with the terminology used in the examination questions (see p. 7).

What you *could* do to help you learn

- Copy selected sections of your notes.
- Summarise your notes into a more compact format, including the key points.
- Create your own flash cards — write key points on postcards (carry them around with you for quick revision during coffee breaks or on the bus).
- Make audio recordings of your notes and/or the key points and play these back.
- Make a PowerPoint presentation of the key points and use this to revise in the last few days before the unit test.
- Discuss a topic with a friend who is studying the same course.
- Try to explain a topic to someone who is not following the course.
- Practise examination questions on a topic.

Approaching the unit examination

Terms used in examination questions

You will be asked precise questions in the examination so you can save a lot of valuable time — as well as ensuring you score as many marks as possible — by knowing what is expected. The most common terms are explained below.

Brief

This means that only a short statement of the main points is needed.

Define

This requires you to state the meaning of a term, without using the term itself.

Describe

This is a request for factual detail about a structure or process, expressed logically and concisely, without explanation.

Discuss

You are required to give a critical account of various viewpoints and arguments on the topic set, drawing attention to their relative importance and significance.

Evaluate

This means that a judgement of evidence and/or arguments is required.

Explain

This means that reasons have to be included in your answer.

Identify

This requires a word, phrase or brief statement to show that you recognise a concept or theory in an item.

List

This requires a sequence of numbered points one below the other, with no further explanation.

Outline

This means give only the main points, i.e. don't go into detail. Don't be tempted to write more than necessary — this will waste time.

State

A brief concise answer, with no reasons, is required.

Suggest

This means that the question has no fixed answer and a wide range of reasonable responses is acceptable.

What is meant by...?

This usually requires a definition. The amount of information needed is indicated by the mark allocation.

The unit examination

When you finally open the test paper, it can be quite a stressful moment. Remember that you must answer *all* the questions on the paper. Read each one carefully and allocate the marks in your mind. Simply writing about the topic referred to in the question will not be enough — you must answer the question.

Some other strategies include:

- *do not* begin to write as soon as you open the paper
- *do* read the questions thoroughly before you start your answers
- *do* identify those questions about which you feel most confident
- *do* answer *first* those questions about which you feel most confident, regardless of order in the paper
- *do read* the question carefully — if you are asked to explain, then explain, don't just describe
- *do* take notice of the mark allocation and try to match this to the number of points you make in your answer
- *do* try to stick to the point in your answer

Time allocation

Do not waste time writing material that will not score marks. Take the following example:

Outline the reasons why an athlete would warm up prior to exercise.   (2 marks)

This is a straightforward question. When it appeared in an examination paper, most students scored the full 2 marks. Many students scored those marks in a couple of sentences and then wasted time writing another half page. Remember, 2 marks means you have to make just two points.

Break the question down

Ask yourself: 'How many things am I being asked to do?' Identify the different parts of the question to ensure that you do everything asked, therefore making it possible to gain all the available marks. Take the following example:

Identify and explain the stages of a warm-up for a sport of your choice.   (6 marks)

This question has 3 marks available for the first part of the question — *identifying* the stages of a warm-up — and 3 marks for the second part of the question — *explaining* the stages of a warm-up.

Plan your answer

Try to be concise, but make sure that you include enough points to match the marks available. Take the following example:

**Identify three responses to exercise. Explain why each response occurs
and state its benefit for the performer.** (9 marks)

This question asks you to:
- identify
- explain why
- state the benefit

It would be easy to write a mini-essay that contains a lot of detailed sports science but fails to answer one or more parts of the question. The question asks for three things, three times. By structuring your answer, you should be able to identify nine points:
- first response
- explain why this response occurs
- state the benefit of this response
- second response
- explain why the second response occurs...and so on

Answer the question set

It is important to answer the question set and not one that you wish had been set. Take the following example:

**Identify the adaptations to, and benefits for, the muscular system
that result from aerobic training.** (3 marks)

Answers relating to the cardiovascular or skeletal systems will waste time and not score any marks.

Content Guidance

This section is a guide to the content of **Unit 1: Participation in Sport and Recreation**. The main areas covered are:

- **Healthy and active lifestyles**
  - development of active leisure and recreation
  - healthy lifestyle
  - effects of exercise — responses and adaptations of the body systems
  - fitness, training and fitness assessment
- **Opportunities and pathways**
  - development of competitive sport
  - performance pathways
  - lifelong involvement
  - long-term athlete development

You may already be familiar with some of the information in these topic areas. However, it is important that you know and understand this information exactly as described in the specification. This summary of the specification content highlights key points and you should find it useful when revising for the Unit 1 exam.

Healthy and active lifestyles

Development of active leisure and recreation

Key points

- **Requirements for participation** — what they are.
- **Recreation and leisure** — definitions, relationships and current trends.
- **Mass participation/Sport for All** — what they mean, why they are pursued and current policies.
- **Contemporary concerns** — what they are, the causes and the effects.

This section introduces the general concepts behind active lifestyles, which are explored in more detail later in the unit.

Requirements for participation

There are four essential requirements: fitness, ability, resources and time.

Fitness

In order to participate in active pastimes safely, and enjoy them, a basic level of fitness is required. However, fitness can be achieved with exercise, so a lack of fitness should not prevent you from taking part. It might slow down your initial involvement until your level of fitness gradually improves.

Ability

Ability refers to your experience and knowledge of the activity and is again essential for participation. Different levels of ability are required for different types of performance. However, many pursuits cater for a wide range of abilities from novice to elite, for different genders and for people with disabilities.

Resources

Resources include the physical equipment necessary to take part, sufficient people to take part with or against, and the money to pay for hire or purchase of facilities and/or equipment. Clearly, without resources, participation is not possible.

Different types of activities require more or less in terms of resources. For example, motor racing and sailing require significant resources compared with walking. The higher up the performance pyramid, the greater the dependence on resources.

Time

Time is essential in order to participate in any type of pursuit. Restrictions on working hours and labour-saving devices mean that we now have more leisure time than ever before. However, our lifestyle often puts a strain on our time and commitments and the wide range of recreational activities available means less time to pursue any particular one.

Concepts of recreation and active leisure

Leisure is time that is free from work, domestic commitments and regular duties or responsibilities. For an activity to be classed as leisure, it must be enjoyable, entered into willingly and voluntarily, and must produce intrinsic rewards for the person involved.

Recreation is the use of leisure time. Recreational activities often involve more physical activity, in contrast to leisure activities, which can be active or passive, for example in the form of **spectatorism**.

We now have more time available (leisure) and greater access and opportunity. However, a shift in social habits means that we are far more sedentary. Consequently our fitness levels and our ability may be perceived to be low — perhaps too low, in our own eyes, to permit participation. This results in less active recreation.

Mass participation and Sport for All

The principle of Sport for All was first established following a campaign in 1972 to highlight the value of sport. This campaign promoted the idea that sport should be accessible to all members of the community and illustrated the benefits to us as individuals and as a society.

In order to encourage more people to take part in sports, initiatives were set up to encourage greater involvement at 'grass roots' level. This refers to sport played at the lowest organised levels.

Contemporary concerns

Contemporary concerns are issues that relate to the present day. Within this context are those issues affecting the health of society, either positively or negatively. Illness and activity levels are the prime focus.

Disorders that are believed to be offset by exercise are called **hypokinetic** disorders.

Obesity

Obesity is a measure of body fat, not weight. A person is classed as obese when his/her body fat level is 25% greater than the recognised norm. The norms are 13–17% for healthy males and 21–25% for healthy females.

Studies show that 22% of men and 23% of women in England are now obese. These figures are predicted to increase to 33% for men and 28% for women by 2010.

Obesity is linked to many problems and diseases, including coronary diseases, diabetes, high blood pressure and certain forms of cancer.

Coronary heart disease

Coronary heart disease (CHD) occurs when the arteries feeding the heart are damaged. Excess cholesterol in the diet attaches to the walls of these arteries in the form of plaque deposits. These deposits restrict the flow of blood through the arteries and contribute to a loss of elasticity of the arteries.

The symptoms of coronary heart disease are hard to detect. The first clear symptom may take the form of a sudden **heart attack** when the disease is at an advanced stage.

The following factors are known to increase the risk of CHD:
- diabetes
- high blood pressure
- high LDL ('bad' cholesterol)
- low HDL ('good' cholesterol)
- menopause
- not getting enough physical activity or exercise
- obesity
- smoking

Diabetes

Diabetes is a condition in which the body is unable to regulate blood sugar levels efficiently in order to prevent hyperglycaemia (blood sugar levels too low for normal bodily functions). This occurs when the body is unable to make sufficient insulin, or when the body becomes resistant to insulin.

If left untreated, diabetes can lead to serious long-term complications such as:
- cardiovascular disease
- chronic renal failure
- retinal damage, which can lead to blindness
- nerve damage (of several kinds)
- microvascular damage, which may cause impotence and poor healing. Poor healing of wounds, particularly of the feet, can lead to gangrene, which may require amputation

High blood pressure

Blood pressure is the force exerted by the blood in the arteries. Every time the heart beats, blood is ejected into the arteries. The greater the volume of blood ejected, and the greater the strength of ventricular contraction, the higher the pressure is in the artery.

There are always two blood pressure readings: **systolic** when the heart contracts and **diastolic** when the heart relaxes.

High blood pressure can cause serious problems such as:
- increasing the risk of heart attack
- angina
- stroke
- kidney failure
- peripheral artery disease (PAD)

High cholesterol

Cholesterol is a liquid fat that binds to proteins. There are two types of cholesterol, HDL and LDL. If there are a lot of proteins present (**high-density lipoproteins** or HDL) then it is good fat; if there are low levels of proteins (**low-density lipoproteins** or LDL) then this is the bad fat.

Cholesterol is essential for bodily function. However, too much LDL cholesterol is dangerous.

Metabolic syndrome

Metabolic syndrome is a combination of medical disorders that increase the risk of cardiovascular disease and diabetes. It is associated with abdominal fat and high blood pressure and is brought about largely by low levels of activity. This in turn leads to increased likelihood of:

- cardiovascular disorders
- blood fat disorders — high triglycerides, low HDL cholesterol and high LDL cholesterol — that foster plaque build-up in artery walls
- insulin resistance or glucose intolerance
- coronary heart disease
- type II diabetes
- hormonal imbalance

Stress

A stress is a stimulus that produces a reaction in the body. Athletes are used to these 'stressors'. They can control them and actually encourage them so that their bodies make physiological changes to enable them to perform better (see the responses to performing a warm-up on pp. 28–29).

However, within the context of this section, stress means a build-up of events or stimuli that cannot be dealt with. The body may have been producing the correct responses to prolonged low levels of stress that have been unresolved. As a consequence, the nervous system may remain slightly activated and continue to pump out extra stress hormones over an extended period. This can weaken the body's immune system, and cause other related health problems such as:

- anxiety or panic attacks
- a feeling of being constantly pressured, hassled and hurried
- irritability and moodiness
- physical symptoms, such as stomach problems, headaches, or even chest pain
- allergic reactions, such as eczema or asthma
- problems with sleeping
- drinking too much, smoking, overeating, or taking drugs
- sadness or depression

Sedentary lifestyles

A sedentary lifestyle is one that is predominantly lacking in physical activity.

Ageing population

In the UK, 16% of the population are aged 65 or over. The population has grown by over 5 million in the past 30 years, an 8% increase. The population of the over-65s grew by 31% over the same period, with a growth of nearly 6% for the over-85s.

Access

In terms of sport and physical activity, access refers to a combination of opportunity and provision.

Many people do not have equal access to sport, often as a result of discrimination owing to cultural variables. A number of target groups have been identified, all of whom have, for a variety of reasons, found it difficult to access sport and recreation.

Opportunity

Cultural or religious factors may provide a barrier to the potential opportunity to groups based on:

- gender
- class
- race
- age
- ability

Provision

Provision relates more directly to facilities and whether these aid or hinder participation.

What the examiners will expect you to be able to do

- Name the basic requirements for participation and explain how they apply to different groups in society.
- Discuss how these basic requirements have affected activity levels up to and including the present day.
- Define and link the concepts of recreation and leisure, stating current trends in both with reasons or justifications for these trends.
- Understand the concept of mass participation/Sport for All, as well as recent policies designed to increase sporting participation at this level.
- Understand what the contemporary concerns are, and the causes and effects of each.

Healthy lifestyle

Key points

- **Health and fitness** — definitions and the differences between the two.
- **Diet** — what makes a healthy diet, the role of the different food groups for health, and how each group needs to be manipulated the more active you are.
- **Energy** — what it is, where it comes from, how much you need; what happens if you have too much or not enough.
- **Balanced lifestyles** — what needs to be balanced and the potential consequences of not getting it right.
- **The effects of ageing** — how it can adversely affect performance and what can be done to minimise these effects.

Health, fitness and exercise

The terms health and fitness may seem to be linked and have many similarities. However, they are quite distinct.

Health is defined as a complete state of physical and mental well-being and not merely the absence of disease or infirmity.

Fitness is defined as the ability to meet the demands of the environment without undue fatigue.

Both terms relate to how well you are able to meet the demands of your environment. In terms of health, your environment is your lifestyle and the requirements that it places upon you. In terms of fitness, your environment is a sport-related one and it depends on the sport you play — and indeed the role that you have within that particular sport.

Exercise is a physical activity that produces a positive physiological adaptation. You may undertake exercise to improve or maintain your health or fitness. The difference is that exercise undertaken to improve fitness is (usually) more specific and invariably at a higher intensity.

Positive benefits to achieving health and/or fitness

The contemporary concerns that can be classed as hypokinetic disorders are identified on pp. 14–16. Clearly, an increased activity level can have significant health benefits.

The most obvious benefit to exercising, or simply increasing your activity levels, is the potential for decreasing body fat levels. However, there are numerous other benefits to the individual, as shown in the table on p. 19.

Physiological benefits of a more active lifestyle	Psychological benefits of a more active lifestyle
Decreased abdominal fat	Increased confidence
Decreased blood pressure	Increased drive
Decreased likelihood of suffering from metabolic syndrome	Increased motivation
Decreased risk of coronary heart disease	A general feeling of mental wellbeing
Decreased risk of high cholesterol	Better able to concentrate and for longer periods
Decreased risk of diabetes	Better able to deal with stress
Better able to offset the ageing process	

Energy expenditure and fat loss

Body fat is needed for insulation and potential energy. In terms of potential energy, 1 lb or 0.45 kg of body fat is the equivalent of 3200 calories. In order to lose body fat you must expend more calories than you consume. However, starvation can have several adverse effects. It can:

- slow down the body's basic metabolic rate
- lead to loss of fluids
- lead to loss of lean muscle tissue

Body fat loss should be achieved by careful manipulation of dietary intake and an increased calorific expenditure. In short, this means a balanced diet and an increase in activity levels.

Basal metabolic rate

Basal metabolic rate (BMR) is the speed at which the body converts and uses calories. People with a high BMR are usually thin, while people with a low BMR usually carry excess weight in the form of fat. Factors that affect BMR include:

- height
- muscle mass
- age
- pregnancy
- smoking
- caffeine
- hormones

BMR - speed at which the body converts and uses calories

Tall people and people with high muscle mass have higher BMRs than shorter people and those with lower muscle mass. BMR decreases after peak physical maturation (from early 30s onwards). BMR increases during pregnancy, and smoking and caffeine increase BMR.

The hormones listed on p. 20 play a part in controlling and elevating BMR.

Growth hormone	Stimulates protein synthesis and growth
Thyroxin	Plays the biggest single role in controlling the BMR (cell respiration) as it stimulates growth and development
Insulin	Stimulates cellular uptake of glucose and the formation of glycogen and fat
Glucagon	Stimulates cellular hydrolysis (breakdown) of glycogen
Epinephrine, norepinephrine	'Fight or flight' hormones cause increases in heart rate, heart output, blood pressure, respiratory rate, metabolic rate
Testosterone	Secreted by the interstitial cells; in males it influences the development and maintenance of the sex organs and development of secondary sex characteristics

One of the keys to successful fat loss is to maintain a high BMR. This can be achieved by:

- eating frequent meals
- exercising

Coronary heart disease and high cholesterol

Increased activity levels can help to combat the effects of both high cholesterol and coronary heart disease.

Fat is a fuel. Low-intensity activities use a greater percentage of calories from fat. If the intensity of the activity is high, the majority of the energy is taken from stored muscle glycogen and not fats. However, increased activity levels are still of benefit because:

- the surges of blood help to flush out the arteries
- fat stores are used post-activity to help fuel recovery and to refuel the muscle glycogen stores

Osteoporosis

Osteoporosis is a disease in which bones become fragile and more likely to break. It is usually experienced by elderly people, with women being at greater risk.

Bone, like most other body tissue, responds to increased activity levels. It responds by laying down new stress lines in the direction of the stress experienced. This increases the density and the strength of the bone.

Type II diabetes

Exercise helps to prevent the onset of non-hereditary diabetes because it combats or offsets many of the factors that can lead to diabetes.

Type II diabetes is more common in people who are prone to putting on excess weight. This can include ethnic groups (due to diet or hereditary body compositions), social groups (again as a result of diet or lifestyle), or age-defined groups (such as the aged population).

Nutrition and weight management

Food groups and a balanced diet

There are seven food groups and these are shown in the table. Carbohydrates, fats and proteins are the energy providers. Vitamins, minerals, fibre and water do not provide energy.

Food group	Main bodily function	Good sources	Notes
Carbohydrates	• High-intensity fuel • Aids the utilisation of fats as an energy source	Foods containing sugars and starch: fruit, pasta, wheat, cereals, chocolate	There are two types of carbohydrate: simple and complex
Fats	• Low-intensity energy • Insulation	Fish, animal and dairy products	There are soluble and insoluble fats
Proteins	• Growth • Repair • 'Last-resort' energy	Meats, soya, dairy products	Proteins are made from amino acids of which there are two types, essential and non-essential
Vitamins	• Required to facilitate physiological functions	Animal and dairy products, fruits, vegetables and grains	There are fat-soluble and water-soluble vitamins
Minerals	• Aid vitamin absorption • Provide the structure for bones and teeth • Essential in many bodily functions	Vegetables, fruits, fish, nuts	Major minerals include calcium, magnesium, potassium and sodium Trace minerals include zinc and fluorine
Fibre	• Essential for healthy bowel function	Plant foods, fruits, vegetables, beans and oats	There are two types of fibre: soluble and insoluble There are no calories, vitamins or minerals in fibre and it is not digested when we eat it
Water	• Involved in almost every bodily function • Primarily seen in its role of thermoregulation and transport	Fruits and water as a drink	

Hydration

Hydration is a term used to describe the state the body is in when it has optimal water content. Dehydration is when water content is low to the point where it is beginning to affect the functioning and efficiency of the body.

Water is essential for the body to function. Every physiological process in the body requires water and our bodies comprise almost two-thirds water.

Losing water

The body loses water in a variety of ways:

- through daily urine output
- through sweating — the hotter the climate, or the more intense and longer the duration of the activity, the more we sweat
- through respiration
- through ventilation, as air has to be moistened as it enters the body

Food pyramid

The foods we eat are classified into seven categories. However, as our lifestyles differ, so do our requirements for the different food groups. We always require a balance of all seven food groups, but circumstances might alter the balance. For example, the dietary demands of a pre-pubescent girl are different from those of a 75-year-old sedentary male, whose requirements are different from those of an elite-performing 28-year-old marathon runner.

To help clarify this situation, various organisations have used the idea behind a food pyramid. The food pyramid shown below is a guide for people aged over 70.

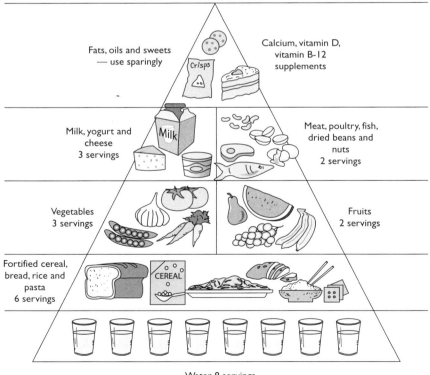

Water 8 servings

Dietary requirements for exercise

Dietary guides look at the requirements to maintain general health. Any activity or change to the norm will mean that the diet has to be modified to take these changes into account. By looking at the role of each of the seven food groups and analysing the activity that you take part in — for example, what type of fuel is required for training, for performing, to adapt to the demands placed on the body by stress such as exercise, how much water and electrolytes you will need to replace — you should be able to plan your diet effectively.

Current trends in health

The health of the population of a country is determined by one or a combination of dietary habits, lifestyle habits, recreation and activity levels.

- Poor dietary habits include a high dependency on processed, sugary, high fat and or dairy foods. It also covers poor food preparation, such as fast foods and those that are deep fried.
- Lifestyle habits include sedentary pastimes, reliance on vehicle transport, alcohol, tobacco and other social drugs, as well as a stressful work environment.
- Recreation habits that contribute to a poor level of health include those that are not physically active. They may relate closely to the poor lifestyle habits above.

If a society has a culture that endorses any of the factors above, then it is likely that there will be severe health issues and concerns.

Contrast the USA and Finland

The lifestyle of many Americans has led to the USA having the highest levels of child and adult obesity. Although sport has a high cultural position, the desire and pressure to win has contributed to many people winning by association — spectating — rather than taking part actively. The USA has for a long time been associated with large portions of quick, mass-produced processed foods. It is little wonder that many 'fat camps' have been established to help people to lose weight.

Poor diet, excessive use of tobacco and alcohol and a lack of physical activity were blamed during the 1980s for Finland having a mortality rate from cardiovascular diseases that was among the world's highest, especially for middle-aged males.

The most common causes of death in Finland were:

- cardiovascular diseases (this was the most common cause)
- respiratory illnesses (at twice the Swedish rate)
- lung cancer (at three times the Swedish rate)
- accidental or violent death (at a frequency 50% higher than the Swedish figure)

However, there has been significant work to improve the situation, as is documented in the Health in Finland Document, May 2006.

Health in Finland

- Public health in Finland has improved rapidly over the past few decades.
- Life expectancy has almost reached the best European figures.

- Mortality from coronary heart disease and stroke has decreased by three-quarters from the world's highest level in the early 1970s.
- There has also been a major reduction in the incidence of many cancers and infectious diseases, oral health has improved and mortality from traffic and work accidents has decreased.
- Furthermore, both perceived health and functional capacity have improved.
- This progress is due to a number of factors related to population structure, living conditions and behaviour.

Dietary habits and nutrition are important determinants of a large number of chronic diseases. The Finnish diet has become much healthier over the past decades.

Regular physical activity promotes health. The proportion of physically active adults has steadily increased, but still only 30–50% of adults are active enough.

Japan offers an illustration of how lifestyle factors directly influence the health of its people.

Two aspects of Japanese culture have recently illustrated significantly different approaches and effects:
- Japan has recently experienced a decrease in activity levels among its populus. Obesity levels have risen significantly, particularly for men, and despite government attempts to help, diabetes levels and cardiovascular disease have shown no improvements.
- Often associated with the high expectations and consequent stresses of adolescence, Japan has one of the world's highest suicide rates among its under 21-year-olds.

In contrast, the Japanese island of Okinawa is described as the 'best place on earth for healthy aging'. The Okinawans have:
- more people over 100 years old per 100 000 population than anywhere else in the world
- the lowest death rates from cancer, heart disease and stroke
- the highest life expectancy for both males and females over 65
- the highest life expectancy in all age groups among females

Contributory reasons for this are:
- eating less food, which produces fewer free radicals
- smoking is not common
- activity levels are high
- diet is naturally low in fats

Balanced lifestyle

A balanced diet can mean different things to different people.

Energy balance
An overweight person wishing to lose body fat needs to consider his/her basic energy requirements (basal metabolism or basal metabolic rate (BMR)) and ensure that he/she does not consume in excess of this.

An active athlete needs to balance his/her energy requirements for performance, consuming not simply the correct *quantity* of calories but the right *type* of calories.

Physical activity can place significant demands on the energy supplies of the body. Working muscles require energy, so the more muscles that are used, the more energy will be required. Bigger muscles require more energy than smaller ones. The intensity at which the muscles are working, and the duration for which they are working, also affect energy usage.

Dealing with stress

The body is designed to deal with stress, and physiological responses enable the body to cope with the stress. However, if the body's responses are engaged without being properly dissipated, this can lead to a feeling of anxiety and unease that can in turn lead to increased heart rate, blood pressure and other related circulatory problems.

The term work–life balance generally refers to the fact that many people spend too much time working, and allocate insufficient time to recreation or leisure. The consequence of this is likely to be an inability to release stresses and a build-up of tension. There is also a tendency in these situations for the over-zealous worker not to allow sufficient time to prepare and eat healthily or to exercise. This results in a potentially unhealthy person with increased risk of illness, and in particular the symptoms associated with metabolic syndrome.

Effects of ageing

Ageing has an effect upon performance, and understanding exactly why this happens is important.

The pre-puberty performance of boys and girls is largely comparable. After puberty, both males and females have an increased capacity for performance and make improvements in that performance. This increased capacity peaks at different ages for different components of fitness.

There has been a long-held belief that for sports that require speed and flexibility, such as gymnastics and track and field events, athletes are past their prime once they cease to be teenagers. On the other hand, athletes competing in events requiring muscular and cardiovascular endurance, such as the marathon and 'iron man' type triathlons, are considered to peak in the mid-30s. However, assumptions and generalisations are dangerous unless they are supported by factual understanding.

Muscular strength

Athletes can lose maximal strength with age for a variety of reasons:
- As we age we might be less active and as a result our muscular system will atrophy.
- There appears to be a degeneration of the nerves supplying the muscles.
- Extra collagen fibres are laid down between the muscle fibres, which reduces the elasticity and flexibility of the muscle, with a resultant decrease in efficiency.

Cardiovascular and cardio-respiratory endurance (lung functioning)

Three main reasons have been given for potential losses in cardiovascular and cardio-respiratory efficiency:

- a decline in maximal heart rate of up to 10 beats per minute per decade
- decreased left ventricular contractile performance resulting in a decreased stroke volume
- a decline in total blood volume, plasma, and red blood cells

Two further reasons are:

- a potentially lower level of alveolar capillarisation
- reduced elasticity of the lungs and respiratory muscles resulting from collagen layers, which produce lower rates of gaseous exchange

Resting metabolic rate (RMR)

RMR tends to decrease as we age because we are likely to become more sedentary and lose muscle mass — two of the biggest factors affecting metabolic rate.

Flexibility

Past activity levels are likely to affect our flexibility as we age.

Factors that affect mobility include:

- wear and tear on connective tissue — ligaments and cartilage
- increased collagen content in skeletal muscle
- scar tissue that may have developed
- loss of muscle elasticity and joint mobility through inactivity or lack of stretching exercises
- reductions in bone density

Age affects athletic performance but regular activity can offset these negatives.

What the examiners will expect you to be able to do

- State the definitions of health and fitness and explain how they can affect each other.
- Understand how to achieve both health and fitness.
- Explain what makes a healthy diet, the role of the different food groups for health, and how each food group needs to be manipulated depending on how active you are.
- Understand what energy is, where it comes from, and how much you need.
- Understand the consequences of having insufficient energy or too much (due to over-eating).
- Understand the term 'balanced lifestyle' and the potential consequences of not getting it right.
- Discuss the effects of ageing and what causes them.
- Understand the role of exercise in minimising the effects of ageing.

Effects of exercise: responses and adaptations of the body systems

Key points

- **Responses and adaptations** — what they are, the differences between the two, how responses and adaptations can benefit the performer, how they can be manipulated.
- **The muscular–skeletal system** — what makes up this system and how the different components respond to and then adapt to exercise.
- **The cardiovascular system** — the components that make up the system, its role in health and fitness, how it responds to and then adapts to exercise, the different types of exercise, and the different types of responses and adaptations.
- **The respiratory system** — what makes up the system and how it functions, how different environments can affect its function, how it responds to and then adapts to exercise and environmental changes.
- **The neuromuscular system** — the link between the brain and resulting muscle contraction, how contractions can vary in the force generated, how the system responds to and then adapts to exercise, and the benefits gained for the athlete.

It is essential that you are familiar with the following terms:
- **anatomy** — the physical structure of the body
- **physiology** — the way the body functions
- **response** — a temporary change that happens quickly
- **adaptation** — a permanent change that takes place over time
- **structural** — describes make-up or anatomy and often relates to a change
- **functional** — describes the way the body works (its physiology) and often relates to a change

It may be helpful to picture the body as a clever but lazy combination of parts, to the extent that it constantly seeks out ways to function with the least amount of effort. Consequently, responses take place that enable the body to function with minimal effort and adaptations occur to enable the body to perform in a now familiar environment without undue stress. For example, adaptations that enable an aerobic athlete to perform better occur so that the body meets the demands made on it with less stress.
- Immediate changes to energy systems during exercise are **responses**.
- More permanent changes as a result of prolonged exposure to a particular type of exercise are **adaptations**.

Activity

Arrange the items in the list on p. 28 into an 'order of events' and then provide an example for each item.

- adaptations
- physiology
- stress
- responses
- functional responses

- types of stress
- anatomy
- structural responses
- structural adaptations
- functional adaptations

Warming up and cooling down

Warming up and cooling down encourage responses, and training encourages adaptations. The general responses that occur as a result of warming up are outlined below.

Stages of warm-up

Stage 1: initial preparation

The aim is to encourage the necessary responses to facilitate improved performance. This is achieved through gross motor skills, using slow, continuous exercise, and increasing in intensity.

The benefits include:
- the release of adrenaline, which results in an increase in heart rate
- increased ventilation, which speeds up oxygen delivery
- heat generation
- speeding up localised muscular metabolism
- dilation of blood vessels
- increased muscle elasticity, which results in greater force and speed of contraction
- decreased muscle viscosity, which results in greater force and speed of contraction, and greater flexibility

Stage 2: injury prevention

The aim is to minimise the risk of injury. This is achieved through stretching — active static, passive static, ballistic, dynamic and proprioceptor neuromuscular facilitation (PNF).

The benefits include:
- reduced risk of injury
- an improvement in tension/tone over a greater length of the muscle, enabling a greater force to be exerted
- a reduction in loss of performance with age
- postural improvements

Stage 3: skill practice

The aim is to strengthen the link between mind and muscle and to improve confidence. This is achieved through practising with a partner or group.

The benefits include:
- improved reaction and response due to the increased frequency of nerve impulses
- improved timing, which minimises the risk of injury

Stage 4: sport specific

This is the final preparation before the performance. It is achieved through practising with a partner or group, with increased intensity and simulation of performance conditions.

The benefits are that:
- confidence is developed
- performance is aided

Cool-down

The warm-up prepares for activity; the cool-down prepares for inactivity and for the next training session.

By gradually reducing the intensity of the activity over approximately 20 minutes, the body is able to start the process of recovery more effectively and quickly.

Cool-down involves performing light, continuous exercise during which the heart rate remains elevated. The purpose is to keep metabolic activity high and blood vessels dilated so that oxygen can be flushed through the muscle tissue, removing and oxidising any lactic acid that remains. This prevents blood pooling in the veins which, if exercise is stopped abruptly, can cause dizziness.

The final part of the cool-down period should involve a period of stretching exercises. It is only after recovery has been completed that future training should be considered.

Muscular–skeletal system

- Muscles are attached to bones by **tendons**.
- At joints, bones are attached to bones by **ligaments**.
- Cartilage assists at joints.
- Muscles can only contract, but there are different types of contraction and muscles can take on several different roles.
- Muscle contraction gives stability, allows movement and produces heat.

All muscles have at least one point of **origin** (where they are anchored to the skeleton) and one point of **insertion**. When a muscle contracts, it pulls on the point(s) of insertion and the bone is pulled towards the point of origin. This happens because muscles are attached to bones by tendons. An example is shown in the diagram below.

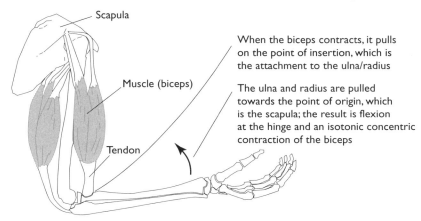

Scapula

Muscle (biceps)

Tendon

When the biceps contracts, it pulls on the point of insertion, which is the attachment to the ulna/radius

The ulna and radius are pulled towards the point of origin, which is the scapula; the result is flexion at the hinge and an isotonic concentric contraction of the biceps

The amount of movement possible is determined by the joint structure and the elasticity of the muscle. Combined, these produce **flexibility**.

Types of skeletal muscle fibre

There are two basic fibre types: **slow twitch** and **fast twitch**. Fast-twitch fibres are subdivided into **type IIa** (**f**ast-twitch-**o**xidative-**g**lycolytic, FOG) and **type IIb** fibres (**f**ast-**t**witch-**g**lycolytic, FTG). Therefore, there are three groups — **type I** (slow twitch), and types IIa and IIb (both fast twitch).

Type I fibres work best with oxygen; type IIb fibres work best when there is insufficient oxygen. Fibres that work best with oxygen must have characteristics that enable them to do so. If fibres are trained for their specific design, then they become even better at working with or without oxygen. For example, when experiencing aerobic training, type IIb fibres will take on the characteristics of type IIa fibres, while type IIa fibres will take on the characteristics of type I fibres.

Work well with oxygen ⟵   Work well when there is insufficient oxygen ⟶

Type I (slow twitch)	Type IIa (FOG)	Type IIb (FTG)
Contract slowly	Contract quicker	Contract quickest
Moderately powerful	Quite powerful	Very powerful
Small	Bigger	Biggest
Many mitochondria	Fewer mitochondria	Very few mitochondria
High myoglobin content	Moderate myoglobin content	Low myoglobin content
Resistant to fatigue	Moderately resistant to fatigue	Easily fatigued
High capillary density	High capillary density	Low capillary density
High aerobic capacity; low anaerobic capacity	Relatively high aerobic and anaerobic capacity	Low aerobic capacity; high anaerobic capacity
Low energy stores (ATP, PC and muscle glycogen)	Higher energy stores	Highest energy stores

Tip If you visualise the three types of fibre on a line from left to right, with type I on the left, type IIa in the middle and type IIb on the right, then all you have to remember is 'left is with O_2' and 'right is without O_2'.

Adaptations to exercise

All three types of fibre adapt to exercise, as summarised in the table below.

Exercise	Type I	Type IIa	Type IIb
Low-intensity, long-duration	Become better able to produce energy aerobically	Start to take on type I characteristics	Begin to become more aerobically efficient
High-intensity, short-duration, repeated with little rest	Take on type IIa characteristics	Become better able to delay lactic acid build-up	Take on type IIa characteristics
High-intensity, short-duration	Begin to become more anaerobically efficient	Start to take on type IIb characteristics	Become better able to produce energy anaerobically

The responses of the skeletal system include responses at the joints and connective tissue. Increasing temperature decreases the viscosity of the synovial fluid and slightly increases ligament elasticity. This aids a greater range of movement.

Regular exercise affects the bones, joints and connective tissue, but not always in a positive way. The bones increase in density and strength as a result of regular stress. This is more obvious as a result of weight-bearing activities, but the continual pull of the muscles on the bone produces similar adaptations. Exercise puts a great demand on the body's calcium stores, which are maintained within the bones. Depletion can lead to bones becoming more brittle and this can become a problem in later life, particularly for women. A good diet is essential to help maintain bone strength.

Weight-bearing activities can also encourage the hyaline cartilage to thicken, therefore aiding the cushioning and smooth movement of bones at joints. However, weight-bearing activities can lead to joint damage, such as cartilage tears or splits, ligament strains, tears or ruptures, and wear and tear to the surfaces of the articulating bones. Therefore, the potential benefits must be weighed against the potential damage.

Cardiovascular system

Before examining how the cardiovascular system responds and adapts to exercise, we need a basic understanding of its components (anatomy) and how it works.

- The heart is a muscular organ that operates within the circulatory system and is central to the cardiovascular system.
- The circulatory system delivers the cells' requirements and removes their waste products.
- The cardiovascular system refers to the ability of the heart, blood vessels and blood to work under stress to deliver the requirements of cells.

You need to know the following key terms:

- **Cardiac output (Q)** is the amount of blood pumped out by the heart/left ventricle in 1 minute. It is equivalent to:
    stroke volume (SV) × heart rate (beats per minute)
- **Stroke volume (SV)** is the volume of blood ejected into the aorta per beat, measured in litres. It is equivalent to:
    end diastolic volume – end systolic volume
- **End diastolic volume** is the volume of blood in the ventricle when it has finished filling.
- **End systolic volume** is the volume of blood remaining in the ventricle after contraction.
- **Venous return** is the amount of blood returned to the heart/right atrium per minute.
- **Bradycardia** is a decrease in resting heart rate below 60 beats per minute.

The heart comprises four chambers, which are made up of a collection of muscles. Two of the chambers are responsible for collecting blood. These are called the atria. The other two chambers are responsible for pumping blood. These are called the ventricles. The heart is divided sagittally by the septum, with an atrium and a ventricle on each side. Both sides of the heart collect and pump blood at the same time, but to different parts of the body — hence the term **dual circulatory system**.

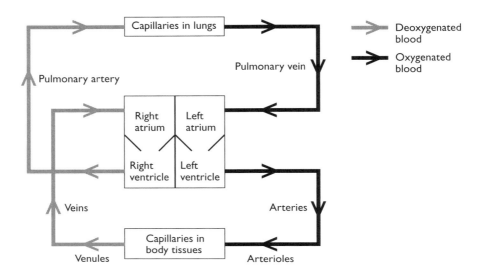

The heart fills up and then empties. The right side of the heart collects *used* blood and sends it to the lungs to be *refreshed*. The left side collects refreshed blood from the lungs and sends it around the body. The better and more efficiently the heart can do this, the greater your potential to perform — particularly if your event requires a lot of oxygen to be delivered over a long period of time.

Oxygen is carried by haemoglobin in the blood. The more haemoglobin in the blood, the greater the body's capacity to transport oxygen.

Blood travels through arteries on its way to the capillaries. The more capillaries there are in the heart, lungs and working muscles, the better the oxygen delivery to them.

Effects of exercise on the cardiovascular system

The diagram on p. 33 shows the effects of exercise on the cardiovascular system.

With regular exercise, the heart becomes stronger and bigger (structural adaptation) and capable of ejecting more blood per beat **(SV)** and per minute **(Q)**, which means that it does not have to beat as often, particularly at rest (bradycardia, functional adaptation).

The arteries retain or even increase their elasticity (structural adaptation), body parts where oxygen is required may experience growth of new capillaries (capillarisation, structural adaptation), vasodilation and vasoconstriction become quicker and more effective (functional adaptation). Consequently vascular shunting takes place more quickly and venous return becomes quicker (functional adaptation).

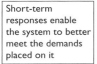

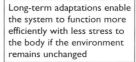

Short-term responses enable the system to better meet the demands placed on it		Long-term adaptations enable the system to function more efficiently with less stress to the body if the environment remains unchanged

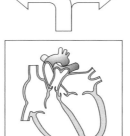

- Increase in stroke volume
- Increase in venous return
- Increase in heart rate
- Increase in cardiac output
- Increase in ventilation rate
- Increase in rates of diffusion
- Increase in blood pressure
- Vascular shunting occurs

- Cardiac hypertrophy
- Increased thickness of ventricular myocardium
- Increased strength of ventricular contractions
- Increased stroke volume
- Increased cardiac output during exercise
- Bradycardia
- Increase in end diastolic volume and decrease in end systolic volume
- Increase in parasympathetic nerve activity
- Increase in red blood and haemoglobin levels
- Increase in alveolar coverage

Respiratory system

The respiratory system is limited in the way in which it can respond to exercise. **Inspiration** and **expiration** are the functional mechanisms, and it is the rate and depth of these two processes that can change. By understanding the mechanics of ventilation, and what each stage is attempting to achieve, you will be better able to appreciate the responses and adaptations that can be made.

A series of causal relationships enables the body to take in and then to expel air.

It is important to understand the concept of a **pressure gradient**. When an area of high pressure exists near to an area of low pressure there is a pressure gradient between them. The greater the difference between the two pressures, the steeper is the pressure gradient. The existence of the gradient means that there will be a transfer of gases between the two areas. The direction is always from an area of high pressure to an area of low pressure, *down* the pressure gradient.

Inspiration

The primary respiratory muscles — the **intercostal muscles** and the **diaphragm** — contract. This causes the chest cavity to increase in volume, which in turn causes the pressure within the lungs to drop. A pressure gradient now exists between the low-pressure area in the lungs and the relatively high-pressure area of the atmosphere. This causes the air to move down the gradient and into the lungs.

Expiration

Relaxation of the intercostal muscles and diaphragm and the **elastic recoil** of the stretched lungs return the thorax to its previous state. This causes an increase in pressure within the lungs. As a result, a new pressure gradient now exists from the lungs to the atmosphere. Air moves down this new gradient, out of the lungs and into the atmosphere. At rest, expiration is largely passive.

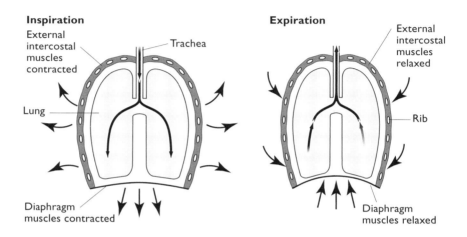

The mechanics of breathing are largely the same at rest as during exercise. However, the ventilation rate is greater and expiration is more active during exercise.

Breathing at rest	Breathing during exercise
Largely passive	Largely active
Expiration is almost entirely passive	Expiration is more active
Breathing is shallow	Breathing is deeper
Breathing is slow	Breathing is faster
Smaller percentage of expired air is CO_2	Greater percentage of expired air is CO_2
Primary respiratory muscles only	Primary and secondary muscles used

The table below illustrates the differences between ventilation at rest and during different intensities of exercise.

Activity level	Ventilation rate
Rest	Approximately 6 litres per minute
Steady-state aerobic exercise	Approximately 80–100 litres per minute in young adult males Approximately 50–80 litres per minute in young adult females
Maximal aerobic exercise	In excess of 120–140 litres per minute

Training does not have a significant effect on lung volumes and capacities. An aerobic training regime can:

- increase the surface area of the alveoli
- strengthen the respiratory muscles and restrict fatigue, which may be experienced towards the end of relatively intense, long-duration activity
- provide small increases in lung volumes — for example, vital capacity (the amount of air that can be forcibly expelled following maximum inspiration) increases slightly, as does tidal volume during maximal exercise

However, such measurements are not used as indicators of aerobic fitness since there is no correlation between lung volume and athletic ability.

VO₂max and factors affecting it

VO₂max is defined as the maximum amount of oxygen that can be taken in and used by the body per minute per kilogram of body weight.

It is believed that a high VO₂max represents the ability to work at a greater intensity before the body begins to rely predominantly on the anaerobic pathways. Consequently, an athlete with a high VO₂max should be able to work harder and be able to sustain that workload for longer.

Athletes frequently focus their training on:

- improving VO₂max
- achieving their potential VO₂max
- being able to sustain work at a higher percentage of their VO₂max

VO₂max refers to oxygen, so many people take the view that they need to target the system responsible for taking in air, namely the respiratory system. However, several factors indicate that this may not be the best option:

- Approximately 75% of the oxygen inhaled is then exhaled. Therefore, taking in more oxygen may not help — we are not able to use that which we have at present.
- Lung capacity can be only marginally increased.

It is therefore the ability to *use* oxygen that has to be targeted. Many of the necessary adaptations are structural and include:

- increased capillarisation of the lungs, which means there will be more blood available to pick up oxygen
- increased numbers of red blood cells and, therefore, higher haemoglobin levels, which will further enable the blood to carry more oxygen
- increased capillarisation in the working muscles, which will enable more oxygen-rich blood to enter the muscle and speed up the removal of carbon dioxide
- increased levels of myoglobin in the working muscles, which will facilitate greater quantities of oxygen becoming available for energy production
- increased numbers of mitochondria, which will enable the muscles to use the extra available oxygen by the aerobic energy pathway
- fat loss, which will mean that the oxygen will not have to be shared by as much body tissue, making more available for the working muscles

Factors that affect VO₂max

Factors that affect VO_2max include:

- age — with increasing age, the heart and lungs begin to lose elasticity, therefore restricting their working capacities
- gender — in men and women of comparable physical stature, women have more body fat and a smaller heart
- body weight — oxygen needs to reach all living cells, so a larger body requires more oxygen
- activity levels — the more regularly the body is exposed to intense aerobic activity, the more likely it is to adapt and improve its aerobic efficiency

Ways of improving aerobic performance

Athletes try to improve their aerobic fitness to levels greater than their competitors' so that they can work harder, longer and recover more quickly.

Traditional aerobic training will improve an athlete's performance. However, in order to be better than the rest, many athletes have sought other ways to achieve improvement.

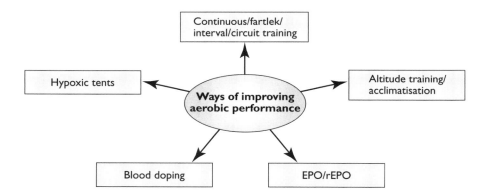

Altitude training

Altitude training is expensive. However, it is probably the most common method used by those who can afford it.

The principle is quite simple. At altitude, atmospheric pressure and the partial pressure of oxygen are lower than at sea level, so there is a lower pressure gradient between the air in the lungs and the atmosphere, and a reduced rate of gaseous diffusion. Consequently, less oxygen arrives at the mitochondria. Therefore, at altitude, an athlete will find it harder to work and train aerobically. The idea is that by training in this environment, the body becomes better able to function with less oxygen, so on returning to a more oxygen-rich environment — sea level — the athlete is able to perform better.

Some points to note

- The sudden increase in altitude leads to a significant drop in aerobic capacity. Therefore, initially, athletes have to reduce their training intensity to compensate.

- The benefits gained may be in part simply due to training intensely in a specific environment — similar to any training camp.
- Oxygen at sea level is of a greater density than at altitude, so the perceived benefits may be lost when the athlete returns to sea level as the body attempts to cope with oxygen of a density greater than at altitude.
- Many athletes are experimenting with training and living at different altitudes — for example, living at sea level and training at altitude (live-low-train-high, LLTH) or living at altitude and training at sea level (LHTL).

Altitude training must be undertaken if the athlete is to perform at altitude. This is known as **acclimatisation** to altitude.

Hypoxic tents

The amount of oxygen in the atmosphere inside a hypoxic tent can be manipulated and controlled. Athletes can live, or in extreme cases even train, in them and simulate the effects of living or training at high altitude. The tents facilitate the LLTH method, allowing athletes the opportunity to experience this type of training without having to leave home. After the initial financial outlay, hypoxic tents become economically more attractive than annual altitude trips.

However, there are drawbacks. First, they are expensive. Second, it can feel strange living and/or sleeping in them and many athletes have complained of headaches and interrupted sleep patterns.

Blood doping

Blood doping is an artificial way of increasing the number of blood cells (particularly red blood cells) in the body. This can significantly increase VO_2max. It is carried out by blood transfusion, using either the athlete's own blood (taken 5–6 weeks previously and suitably stored) or matched blood from another person.

Blood doping is contrary to the ethics of sport and is dangerous. It can lead to:
- increased blood viscosity
- elevated blood pressure
- increased risk of heart failure, stroke and thrombosis
- kidney damage
- infection
- circulatory system overload — the direct result of more blood in the circulatory system than there should be, which means that when vascular shunting takes place, blood pressure increases

EPO and rEPO

EPO (erythropoietin) is a hormone that stimulates the production of red blood cells in bone marrow. It is a blood protein produced primarily in the kidneys during periods of **hypoxia**. (Hypoxia is a condition in which there is an insufficient supply of oxygen to the respiring muscles.)

Athletes who expose themselves to low-oxygen saturation, for example by altitude training, can experience a six- to nine-fold increase in EPO production. This results in the production of more red blood cells and increases oxygen-carrying capacity.

Some athletes have taken advantage of this by using genetically engineered EPO — rEPO, recombinant erythropoietin — and raising their red blood cell levels artificially. This gives an unfair advantage and is potentially dangerous. It can result in:

- increased blood viscosity
- elevated blood pressure
- an increased risk of heart failure, stroke and thrombosis

Note that rEPO is a banned substance.

Neuromuscular system

The efficiency of the muscular system depends on nerve impulses. The neuromuscular system links the brain and the muscles. The central nervous system is the route by which nerve impulses travel.

All muscles in the body are represented along the central nervous system at motor neurone pools. The motor neurones of a particular muscle collect neural impulses that are sent to it, and then rapidly send them to the muscle fibres. If the resulting neuromuscular transmission — called an action potential — is strong enough to reach the muscle fibres, then these fibres will contract maximally.

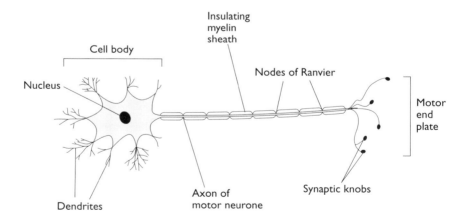

The skeletal muscles are made up of three different types of fibre (see p. 30). As the brain sends messages to the muscles it attempts to recruit first the slow-twitch fibres because they have the lowest threshold, i.e. they require the least stimulation to produce a contraction. As the impulse intensity increases, so the FOG and eventually the FTG fibres are recruited.

If the exercise duration is extended, the slow-twitch fibres may fatigue and be unable to produce the required force. When this happens other fibre types are recruited. The body will need to recruit more motor units to generate the same force that was provided by fewer units at the beginning of the exercise.

The neuromuscular system responds and then adapts to exercise so that messages can be sent more quickly and frequently and so that muscle fibres can be recruited more effectively.

What the examiners will expect you to be able to do

- Understand the differences between a response and an adaptation.
- Understand the difference and the relationship between structural and functional responses.
- Explain how to control the responses and adaptations to maximise performance.
- Describe the short-term and long-term effects of exercise on the muscular–skeletal system, the cardiovascular system, the respiratory system and the neuromuscular system.

Fitness, training and fitness assessment

Key points

- **Components of fitness** — what the different components are, definitions of each, and how to apply them to different sporting events.
- **Methods of fitness training** — the different types of training, the benefits and drawbacks of each type, their suitability to particular fitness benefits, responses and adaptations.
- **Principles of training** — what they are and how to apply them effectively to control the adaptations that you require.
- **Appropriateness of programmes to differing clients** — how and why different groups of people require training programmes that are adapted specifically to their status and needs.
- **Rationale of fitness assessment** — how and why to test, different types of tests, and issues involved in testing.
- **Protocols of recognised fitness tests** — the names of tests for the components of fitness and the specific protocols of each.

Components of fitness

Fitness means different things to different people. The ability to run for a long time is often the benchmark people use to identify 'how fit they are'. Cardiovascular endurance (which would enable an athlete to run for a long time) is only one component of fitness and is not the definitive component for all athletes.

Fitness is perhaps best defined as being able to meet the specific demands of a particular sporting environment without undue fatigue. There are many different types of sporting environment. This means that the demands placed upon athletes also differ. For example, a shot-putter competes in a different environment from a 1500-metre swimmer. Consequently, the athletes have different fitness demands and, therefore, place greater importance on different fitness components.

Physical fitness

Some components of physical fitness are given in the table below. Each component is defined and an example of a sport for which it would be important is given.

Component of fitness	Definition	Sport
Strength — maximal	Ability to exert a maximal force once	Weightlifting
Strength — dynamic	Ability to exert a significant force over a short period of time	2000 metre rowing
Localised muscular endurance	Ability to perform repeated muscular action	Cycling (e.g. Tour de France)
Static strength	Ability to exert a force at a fixed point	Crucifix balance in gymnastics
Cardiovascular endurance	Ability of the body to supply the requirements to, and remove waste from, working muscles over an extended period of time	Marathon
Aerobic capacity	Equivalent to aerobic fitness/power and assessed by measuring VO_2max	10 000 metre
Anaerobic capacity	The length of time that maximal intensity can be sustained	Sprint cycling
Flexibility	Movement at a joint	All sports
Speed	How quickly the body or a body part can be moved	Javelin (pulling the throwing arm through)
Body composition — mesomorph	Predisposition to retaining muscle mass	Sprint
Body composition — ectomorph	Tall, with a predisposition to a small body mass	High jump
Body composition — endomorph	Predisposition to storing body fat	Sumo wrestling

Skill fitness

Some components of skill fitness are given in the table below. Each component is defined and an example of a sport (or sportsperson) for which it would be important is given.

Component of fitness	Definition	Sport/sportsperson
Power	Strength × speed	Shot put
Reaction time	Time taken to act upon a stimulus	Goalkeeper in hockey or football

Component of fitness	Definition	Sport/sportsperson
Dynamic balance	Controlling the centre of gravity while moving	Beam work in gymnastics
Static balance	Controlling the centre of gravity while stationary	Netball goalkeeper defending a shot
Coordination	Ability to link movements together in sequence	Tennis (e.g. the serve)
Agility	Changing direction at speed and with control	Winger in rugby
Strength Maximal	Greatest force to be exerted once	Weight lifter
Dynamic	Exerting a significant force for up to 4 minutes	200 m rower or 800 m runner
Endurance Cardiovascular	Ability of the body to supply oxygen to and remove waste from working muscles for an extended period (up to 720 minutes	Marathon runner
Localised muscular	Ability of a muscle to exert a repeated force for an extended period of time	Tour de France cyclist
Flexibility	Range of movement at a joint	Gymnast

Methods of training

Continuous training

Continuous methods of training work on developing endurance and therefore stress the aerobic energy system. Continuous training involves maintaining the training intensity. Central to this method of training is the performance, at a steady rate or low intensity, of rhythmic exercise that uses the large muscle groups. This should be continued for between 30 minutes and 2 hours.

The health-related benefits of continuous training have been well documented and this, coupled with the fact that little equipment is required in order to participate, has made this method of training one of the most popular among people seeking to improve general health and fitness.

Fartlek (speedplay) training

Fartlek training is often thought of as a modified method of continuous training. It is a form of endurance conditioning in which the aerobic energy system is stressed because of the continuous nature of the exercise. However, unlike continuous training, the intensity of the activity is varied, so both the aerobic and anaerobic systems are stressed. Fartlek sessions are usually performed with the activity ranging from low-intensity walking to high-intensity sprinting.

This type of training can be individualised. The athlete can determine the speed and intensity of the session. Since both aerobic and anaerobic systems are stressed, a wealth of sportspeople can benefit. It is particularly suited to those activities that involve a mixture of aerobic and anaerobic work, for example field games, such as rugby, hockey and football.

Interval training

This is a method of training in which exercise (work) is interrupted by a period of rest (interval) and then repeated. The training session is arranged around a work-to-rest ratio (W:R). An example of a work-to-rest ratio can be taken from a football match, which has two 45-minute work periods and a 15-minute rest interval. The ratio is written as:

W:R = 45:15 or 3:1

The rest period has to be long enough to enable the body to recover sufficiently to be able to perform the next work period at the desired level of intensity and/or the appropriate length of time. Too little rest will prevent the training session from having the desired effect. The type of energy pathway used and the level of energy depletion experienced determine the amount of rest time needed to replenish the pathway fully.

Circuit training

Circuit training consists of a series of exercises arranged in order and designed to develop general body fitness or specific sport-related fitness and skills.

Fixed-load circuits

Each individual begins a circuit and tries to complete a number of laps or repetitions within a time limit.

Individual-load circuits

For example, each individual is tested on each exercise to find the maximum number of repetitions completed in 1 minute. These repetition numbers are then halved to give the number that must be completed per lap. In each session, each individual performs three laps, trying to improve his or her time.

Advantages of circuit training

The great advantage of circuit training is that it can be used to develop strength, power, local endurance, agility, and both anaerobic and aerobic capacities (depending on the exercises chosen) in a limited time and space. Furthermore, large numbers of participants can be involved.

Overload is achieved in circuit training by:
- reducing target times
- increasing exercise resistance (difficulty of the exercise)
- increasing the number of repetitions

Weight-training

During weight-training, subjects perform a series of resistance exercises designed to develop the fitness component they require in specific sport-related muscles.

Weight-training is a predominantly anaerobic activity, although by varying the intensity and duration of the training sessions it can be manipulated to provide numerous benefits, such as muscular strength, endurance, speed, power, body shaping, fat loss, weight gain or loss, muscle tone and improved posture.

When training with weights, it is usual to target specific muscles, muscle groups or body parts. This might involve:
- isolation exercises — working one specific muscle, e.g. leg extension works the quadriceps
- compound exercises — working muscle groups, e.g. the squat works all the main muscles of the trunk and the lower body

Weight-training should not be confused with weightlifting.

Plyometrics and power training
Power is determined by the force exerted by the muscle (strength) and the speed at which the muscle shortens. It has been established that muscles generate more force in contraction when they have been previously stretched. Plyometrics enables this to happen by taking the muscle through a forced eccentric (lengthening) phase before a powerful concentric (shortening) phase. Exercises that might form part of a plyometrics session include bounding, hopping, leaping, skipping, depth jumps (jumping onto and off boxes), throwing and catching a medicine ball, and press-ups with claps.

Aerobic/anaerobic
This refers to the intensity at which you train, for example if you train at a medium to low intensity and the demand for energy can be met through oxygen uptake then the training will be aerobic. If the intensity demands more energy than you can make with oxygen at that given time then you will be working anaerobically.

Speed training
When speed is referred to as maximum speed then the training has to reflect this. Short duration maximum intensity intervals are often associated with speed training. 'Overspeed' training is often used now, e.g. sprinting down hills or using elasticated harnesses to simulate faster movements than the body can generate naturally.

Cross training
This is not a specific method of training, but rather a combination of other training methods. The idea is that it prevents boredom, physiological plateaus and also helps to reduce the likelihood of DOMS (delayed onset of muscular soreness).

Core stability
This type of training emphasises the need to strengthen the muscles that make up the core of the body. The muscles of the abdominals and erector spinae will often work isometrically while performing a role as synergists to the body, thus allowing movements to take place.

Speed, ability and quickness (SAQ)
This type of training makes use of agility ladders, harnesses and resistance equipment in order to develop faster and more efficient neuromuscular links and movements.

Stretching

Stretching is certainly the best way of maintaining or improving muscle elasticity. Performing stretching during a cool-down is an excellent way of maintaining elasticity while aiding recovery.

The different modes of stretching are:
- static — the muscle is taken to its limit and held under tension
  - active static involves the performer stretching the body part
  - passive static is when the performer allows a partner to move the limb to the point of stretch
- ballistic — momentum is used to force the fibres to stretch over a greater range
- PNF — the muscle is stretched to its limit and then undergoes an isometric contraction while stretched; the muscle is relaxed and the process is repeated
- dynamic — the muscle is stretched through a range of movements

The value of pre-activity stretching is currently topical. Performing static stretching in preparation for more sport-specific stretching in a warm-up is almost certainly good practice. However, what is considered dubious is carrying out a few static stretches before embarking upon a particularly ballistic activity, such as trampolining or high hurdling.

Principles of training

Specificity

Fitness is specific to the type of exercise being performed. Training should involve the muscles and energy systems, together with the skills, needed for a particular sport. For example, strength training develops muscular strength; speed training develops fast-twitch muscle fibres and the anaerobic energy systems for stronger, faster movements.

Progression and overload

Progression

Progress should be visible. It might be indicated by performance or by regular fitness tests and should be further documented in the athlete's training diary.

Progression will take place as a result of a gradual increase in training.

Overload

Adaptations are made by the body as a result of the body systems being stressed. For further adaptations to occur, training must be made harder to stress the systems further. This is the principle of progressive overload and should govern all training exercises.

For improvements to occur, the athlete must train at an intensity greater than his or her existing capacity, so that the training load exceeds that to which the body is accustomed. The result of this will be physiological adaptations to the body. Such improvements generally occur as a result of a sustained period of training over several weeks or months.

The relationship between progression and overload

Although overload and progression are similar and depend upon each other, progression is usually associated with an increase in training *volume* while overload is usually associated with an increase in training *intensity*.

Recovery

This is the anabolic state required by the body so that it can replenish, repair and grow. Only after this phase has been completed will the benefits of training be realised. Training at different intensity levels requires different recovery times.

Reversibility

All the physiological adaptations caused by training are reversible if the athlete stops training. For instance, the increase in muscle size (**hypertrophy**), which is a result of strength training, is reversible. If training ceases, the muscle size gradually decreases (**atrophy**). This is a result of the lack of stress to the muscular system.

This principle — which is sometimes referred to as 'regression' or the 'de-training effect' — is true for all training adaptations, including speed and endurance, as well as strength.

Thresholds

These relate to what is known as the FITT principle. The letters FITT represent:
- **F**requency — how often you train
- **I**ntensity — how hard you train
- **T**ime (duration) — how long a training session lasts
- **T**ype — the method of training used

Over-training

Over-training occurs when the recovery (anabolic) phase has not been completed before the next training session.

Training regimes without sufficient in-built recovery intervals may prove to be harmful, rather than beneficial, to the athlete. They can lead to regression and/or injury. Repeated exhaustive exercise can lead to a depressed immune system, and injuries to joints can occur as a result of muscular fatigue.

Therefore, effective training involves the athlete training at an appropriate intensity and duration, with adequate recovery intervals in the programme.

Over-training can be caused by a lack of rest, poor diet (insufficient proteins or carbohydrates) or over-use of intense or maximal training.

Appropriateness of programmes to differing clients

Programmes for different clients

All training programmes need to make full consideration of the individual needs of the person for whom it has been designed. Consequently, it is not advised that anybody's programme is copied. However, certain characteristics are shared by different groups as explained on p. 46.

The young/elderly

For younger people, due consideration must be given to the fact that bones and soft tissue will not be fully developed and so will not be able to withstand the same repetitive stress training that an adult can.

Physical training should avoid high impact exercises such as plyometrics, it should be sub-maximal in nature and also consider that thermoregulation is not as efficient.

As we age, our recovery times from high intensity activity will be longer and so training will have to be less frequent. Progression will need to be applied more gradually, with care being taken when overloading. Slow-twitch fibres seem to show the least effect of aging, so sub-maximal longer duration activities might be better suited. However, this needs to be planned with careful consideration of the potential damage of frequent high-impact training sessions such as running.

Trained/untrained

Trained athletes are able to train more frequently than other people as their recovery times are the fastest. Overload can often be applied at a rate of 5% per week without fear of overtraining.

Trained athletes can spend time making finite adjustments to technique that is probably already of a high standard. They can sustain longer and more frequent bouts of high, near maximal exertion training sessions.

Untrained athletes need to progress gradually and build up to more frequent training sessions, particularly at first. Technique sessions are important but they should focus on the main aspects of a given technique. Exercises are more whole body ones that focus on gross motor skills.

Active and sedentary and healthy/unhealthy

It is likely, although not always the case, that an active person is healthier than a sedentary person.

The sedentary person needs to ensure that it is safe to embark on a programme of physical activity. Intensity levels should be established at a low level, with many frequent but attainable targets set to boost confidence and maintain enthusiasm. It is important that exercise levels and frequencies are set at the minimum level to begin with and gradually increased as progress is made.

The active person has more natural energy and a higher tolerance of training or exercise-related discomfort, so although training frequency and intensity must be monitored, this person would be expected to progress at a faster rate than his/her sedentary counterpart.

Planning to improve

In order to plan an effective training programme, you must:
- decide which components of fitness are needed (analysis of the sport)
- ascertain current levels of fitness against those required (fitness test)
- select the appropriate exercises (methods of training)

- plan when and how to perform the exercises (apply the principles of training)
- review progress (fitness test)

Rationale of fitness assessment

Tests will either be maximal or sub-maximal in nature. Maximal tests — such as the NCF Multistage Fitness test, the 30m flying speed test, the Wingate Anaerobic capacity test — take the athlete to his/her maximum fitness level within the component being measured.

The advantage of a maximal test is that the data received are relatively summative. How the data are used, however, might increase their validity, e.g. the 12-minute Cooper test is a maximal test, measuring the distance covered by an athlete during a 12-minute period. This information needs no interpretation or assumptions. However, the distance can then be used to cross-reference with the aid of a table in order to predict the VO_2max of the athlete. This is a predictive score and so is not as valid as the first data obtained.

Sub-maximal tests, such as the Harvard step test, rely on heart rate data to make predictions based on the information already received. The Harvard step test makes assumptions based on the fact that:
- a steady-state heart rate is obtained for each exercise workload
- a linear relationship exists between heart rate, oxygen uptake and workload
- the maximal heart rate for a given age is predictable
- the biomechanical efficiency of the physical activity performed (i.e. oxygen uptake at a given workload) is the same for everyone

While not being as accurate as maximal tests, sub-maximal tests have the advantage of avoiding the risks and not requiring the athlete to work to exhaustion.

Technology is used to increase the validity and reliability of a fitness test. An example would be when looking at two tests used to measure VO_2max.

The NCF multistage fitness test uses little equipment and as such is a predictive test. The gas analysis test measures the relative volumes of oxygen inspired and expired during progressive maximal exercise in order to provide an accurate result.

Fitness testing is undertaken before, during and after completion of a training programme. It provides a great deal of information, which can be used for a number of purposes — for example:
- identifying areas of strength and weakness in the performer
- providing baseline data for monitoring performance
- identifying strengths and weaknesses in training techniques and practices
- assessing the value of different types of training and helping to modify training programmes
- predicting physiological and athletic potential
- drawing comparisons with previous fitness levels and those of other similar athletes

- ascertaining whether an athlete is capable of competing at a particular level
- enhancing motivation
- forming part of the educational process

Issues to consider before testing

There are issues that must be considered before undertaking any type of fitness test:

- The **validity** of the test — are you aware of the specific areas of fitness that you wish to investigate? If so, is the chosen test valid?
- The **protocol** of the test — are you fully aware of how to run the test accurately?
- The **reliability** of the test — for a test to be worthwhile, it *must* be reliable. The athlete must be able to repeat it several times so that comparisons can be made. The athlete and coach must be confident that the only variable that will have an effect on the result of the test is the fitness of the athlete.
- The **current state of the athlete** — is the athlete equipped for the test, both mentally and physically? Has a physical activity readiness questionnaire (PARQ) been completed?
- **Informing the athlete** — is the athlete fully aware of the test that is about to be undertaken, and has consent been given?

Protocols of recognised fitness tests

Note: Understanding the various fitness tests assumes knowledge of the different components of fitness and how they are defined (see below and pp. 39–41).

Ideally, you should be aware of an appropriate test for each component of fitness. There are many different tests for the various components, and the fitness tests identified here are not exclusive. They are appropriate for the component of fitness in a generic context, but not necessarily for a particular sport.

Appropriate tests for the components of fitness

Maximal strength

Maximal strength is defined as the ability to exert a maximal force once.

Fitness test: 1-rep maximum strength

Protocol: The chosen weight-training exercise is performed for one complete repetition with correct technique and without undue straining.

Localised muscular endurance

Localised muscular endurance refers to the ability of a muscle to perform an action repeatedly.

Fitness test: NCF (National Coaching Foundation) abdominal-conditioning test, which requires athletes to perform sit-ups in time to a pre-recorded tape

Protocol: in a bent-leg sit-up position with arms crossed across the chest, the athlete sits up and down in time to the beeps on the tape.

Flexibility

The movement at a joint is determined by joint structure and muscle elasticity.

Fitness test: sit and reach

Protocol: the athlete sits with legs out-stretched in front and the soles of the feet held flat against a vertical surface. Slowly he/she bends forwards and reaches out with both hands, holding the furthest distance possible.

Speed
This is how quickly a body part and/or the whole body can be moved.

Fitness test: 30-metre sprint

Protocol: allowing a rolling start, the time taken to cross a distance of 30 metres is recorded.

Body composition
Body composition refers to the body mass index ratio — the relative percentages of muscle and fat.

Fitness test: skinfold callipers

Protocol: on the left side of the body, measurements (in mm) are taken at the following sites: biceps, triceps, subscapular and suprailiac. The results are totalled and recorded. The values measured can be compared with a 'norm model' to provide a relative body fat level.

Power
> power = strength × speed

Fitness test: sergeant jump

Protocol: First measure the maximal vertical standing reach. The athlete then jumps as high as possible from a standing position. The difference between the reach height and the jump height is recorded. The difference between the two heights is proportional to the power generated, assessed from standard tables.

What the examiners will expect you to be able to do

- Identify the components of fitness with appropriate definitions and apply each to different sporting events, and also to your own sporting event.
- Explain what a method of training is, and understand the different methods of training, the characteristics of each, and the components of fitness that each can develop, as well as the advantages and disadvantages of each method.
- Describe the different principles of training and how to apply them effectively to control the adaptations required.
- Understand why training programmes need to be different for different people, and adapt programmes specifically to different requirements.
- Understand how and why testing is done, and discuss different types of tests and issues that might arise when testing.
- Describe the different protocols of recognised fitness tests for the main components of fitness and the validity and reliability of each test.

Opportunities and pathways

Development of competitive sport

Key points
- The role that early sports **festivals** played in the historical development of sport.
- The impact that the **Industrial Revolution** had on life in nineteenth-century Britain and the effect this had on the development of **rational sport**.
- The development of the Olympic Games and the issues that have affected the Games.
- The increasing **commercialisation** and **Americanisation** of sport in the twentieth and twenty-first centuries.
- How the increasing extrinsic rewards in sport have led to a corresponding rise in **deviance**.

Festivals of sport

Historical development of sport
The Greeks and the Romans established the first sporting festivals as celebrations, as well as to prepare the men for fighting.

Most early sports were used to prepare for war or to develop hunting skills, and so are referred to as combat sports. The Norman Conquest of 1066 formed a new social order in England, creating a landed gentry and a subservient peasant class. Combat sports followed this division. This was a period of instability and war, and there was a need for all men to maintain their fighting fitness.

The young gentry were the knights — an elite band who spent years developing their fighting and horsemanship skills to fulfil this honour. The main focus for their sporting training was the joust and the tournament.

Archery was a requisite military skill for the lower classes. The longbow was an essential part of English military strategy. A succession of English kings made it compulsory for all men to own a bow and to practise on Sundays.

Festival games and popular recreations
During the pre-industrial period, the time available for sport was often restricted to holy days. Travel was difficult and so recreation activities were local and used ready-to-hand materials. Recreation activities changed through the year. In the winter, mass games such as mob football were played. These were often violent contests with few rules. In the summer, gentler, more individual and athletic-type activities were followed.

The year began with spring fertility festivals, although some games took place as early as New Year's Day and Plough Monday (the first Monday after Christmas). Most, however, focused on Easter. Shrove Tuesday was a particularly popular day for violent mob games, especially forms of football. May Day was often marked by games in which young men chased women, again concerned with rituals of fertility. Whitsuntide was the high point of the sporting year, with much dancing and games. This was a slack time for agriculture, and crops and animals were left to grow. Summer games tended to be gentler — running, jumping and throwing contests. The church provided space to play, often offered patronage to games and festivals, and may have donated prizes.

The modern Olympic Games

The Olympic Games originated in Ancient Greece. They began as funeral games, and were held every 4 years as part of a religious ceremony to the god Zeus. Many of the rules and regulations of the ancient Games can be seen in the modern version, which are still held every 4 years.

During the later part of the nineteenth century, a number of people, including Dr Penny Brookes and Baron Pierre de Coubertin, began to work towards reintroducing the Olympic Games. The first modern Games were held in Athens in 1896. De Coubertin hoped the Games might help prevent war and would develop international friendship. Sportsmanship was central to the Games.

The Olympic Games are now organised by the International Olympic Committee, which chooses the host city and coordinates the huge amounts of money necessary to put on the Games. Most of the IOC's income comes from selling the festoon (the five-ring logo) to multinational sponsors and from media rights.

For most of the twentieth century the Olympics was an amateur event — all the performers competed purely for enjoyment, and although the winner received a medal, it had no monetary value. However, as the Games moved into the second half of the twentieth century, television coverage opened up a huge global audience, making the Games attractive to commercial sponsors.

Most of the credit for this reliance on commercial funding goes to Peter Uberroth, who led the organising committee for the 1984 Los Angeles Olympic Games. Owing to the security problems of the 1972 Munich Games and the bankruptcy of the Montreal Games in 1976, both the US federal government and the California state government withdrew funding in the run up to the 1984 Games. This left Uberroth with the dilemma of how to find the money to pay for the Games. His answer was to offer the television rights to just one company, and to sell the festoon to commercial sponsors. This proved to be a major success; not only did Uberroth raise enough money to pay for the Games, but for the first time they actually made a profit. The 'Hamburger' Games, as they became known due to the overt profile given to the sponsors (and in particular McDonald's), created the model for the organisation and funding of future global Games.

The presence of the media has turned sport into a commodity that can be bought and sold. Television companies pay huge amounts of money to cover sports; and advertisers and sponsors back sport because of the exposure they will get in the media. Individual athletes train and prepare for sport in the knowledge that the media will give them a stage on which to present their talents — and also gain wealth.

The pressure of being able to train and compete at the highest level made its demands on athletes in terms of time and expense. This led in the 1970s to the concept of **shamateurism**, which in turn led to a change in emphasis in sport with the 'win' ethic replacing the 'recreational' ethic. To many performers, sport had become a career rather than a leisure pursuit. Commercial pressures increasingly permeated all sports. By 1981 the IOC had removed the term 'amateur' from the Olympic Charter.

The Olympics receives most of its funding from US television networks, which pay in excess of $400 million for the exclusive rights to screen the Olympic Games. This kind of financial influence gives the television companies control over many factors. For example, we are now used to having to stay up late to see key events such as the 100m final, so that it fits with the prime time television slot on the east coast of the USA.

International sports festivals

At the start of the twentieth century, most of the popular sports established international sports bodies, which began to organise international fixtures and competitions. These tended to be run either with a festival approach where countries play in a series of games and events over a period of up to 3 weeks, or with a knockout format where rounds are played and the winning team progresses to the next round.

The big events, such as the FIFA World Cup and the Commonwealth Games, are now run on a similar pattern to the Olympics — every 4 years. Other events, such as the IAFF Athletics and the Cricket World Cup, are run on a shorter rotation. Like the Olympics, all international sports festivals rely on funding from sponsors and media rights.

What the examiners will expect you to be able to do

- Discuss the importance of the link between combat sports and the need to prepare for war in pre-industrial Britain.
- Explain how early sports were divided by social class and background.
- Explain the importance of the church and the local gentry in the organisation of festival games.
- Discuss how the modern Olympic Games are a combination of ancient and modern festivals.

Tip You should be able to describe and use at least two different popular recreations in your answers.

Impact of the Industrial Revolution and the emergence of rational sport

After the Industrial Revolution, most people lived and worked in urban areas and the influence of the rural elements from the popular recreation era steadily declined. (Modern sport is also urban sport.)

There were a number of changes in the way people lived and worked that had an influence on sport in the post-industrial period:

- **Urbanisation** meant large populations moving into cities and towns where there was a lack of space for recreation.
- **Industrialisation** led to life based around the factory system and machine time. The old saints' days and holy days were largely lost and work was no longer organised around the seasons — every week was a busy time.
- **Working conditions** initially were very poor for the lower classes, with long shifts and little free time. The twentieth century saw a gradual increase in free time: legislation brought in the Saturday half day, the 10-hour Act, and early closing for shop workers.

Economics characterised by the systems of capitalism and industrial patronage led to the formation of works and church teams, which often developed into professional clubs. Sport had become part of the entertainment business and many entrepreneurs saw that money could be made from it.

The development of rationalised sport began in public schools and was spread by 'old boys', church men and school masters working in local communities. Active and manly recreational activities were seen as a means of social control, keeping both schoolboys and the working classes out of trouble while at the same time developing skills and virtues that would be useful to the ever-expanding empire.

Codification

Organised games began to appear in public schools (attended by boys from the upper classes), at first as spontaneous recreations and for the most part disapproved of by the teachers. However, as the games became more developed it was recognised that educational objectives could be passed on through participation in games. Sports became a feature of all public schools, with team games forming the central core. The main sports were football and cricket (and rowing at schools situated near rivers). These games were physically strenuous and demanding. They relied on cooperation and leadership — all characteristics that a gentleman needed to acquire.

The Industrial Revolution created a new affluent social class (the middle class), resulting in a huge market for private education. Middle-class families wanted their sons to be educated as gentlemen and to service this need there was a huge increase in the number of preparatory schools. Sport became a central part of these new schools.

The development of sport through the public school system of the nineteenth century had a profound effect on the spread of sport throughout society, both in Britain and the British empire. It sowed the seeds of rationalisation, in which sports were codified and regulated by governing bodies. The boys who left the schools spread the cult of manly games across the world.

Codification involved the creation and maintenance of a set of national rules. The developing transport system meant that teams and individuals could travel out of their local areas to compete on a national scale. This highlighted the problem of local versions of games and local rules. In most cases, each sport appointed a national governing body (NGB), which standardised the rules for the sport. The NGBs then began to develop more regular fixtures and competitions.

An effective way of memorising this impact is the mnemonic CAT PUICCA.

- C — **colonial**. Many former public school boys took up posts in the colonial service, helping to administer and govern the empire's colonies. Initially they played among themselves, but gradually introduced the sports and games to the indigenous populations.
- A — **army**. Another career for many old boys was as commissioned officers in the armed forces. Initially the officers used sports as a recreation to fill the long hours, but the social control and moral value of keeping the working-class soldiers occupied were not lost on them. This played an important part in spreading the cult still further.
- T — **teaching**. Many former pupils became teachers, especially in the now expanding preparatory and grammar schools. Often they simply repeated the programme of games and physical recreation they had followed in their school days.
- P — **patronage**. Supporting sporting events and competitions, for example by providing funding for trophies or land for pitches, was another important role undertaken by old boys.
- U — **university**. Cambridge and Oxford (chiefly) gave young men further time and resources to pursue and refine sporting activities. One major problem, though, was the plethora of different rules for the various games. In order to allow everyone to play, compromise rules were required and this was the first step towards the rationalisation of sport.
- I — **industry**. Once they had finished school, many boys returned to their fathers' factories and businesses. Their love of sport needed an outlet and soon clubs were set up which were linked to these factories. At first there were some social limits — only managers and office staff could join the teams — but gradually the lower classes were also admitted.
- C — **church**. Much of the boys' education was based on religion and many took up careers in the church. Muscular Christianity promoted the use of sport for teaching morals and Christian virtues. Many clergymen used it in its most practical form, encouraging sports and setting up teams both in the UK and abroad.
- C — **clubs**. The first stage for many old boys was to form clubs so they could continue to play their games. The Old Etonians is a good example of this type of club.
- A — **administration**. When their playing days were over, many men joined governing bodies and developed their sports by helping to formulate national rules.

What the examiners will expect you to be able to do

- Discuss the impact of the Industrial Revolution on sport.
- Explain what is meant by the term codification.

- Explain why there was a need for national governing bodies in sport.
- Explain the role that Cambridge and Oxford universities played in the development of sport.

Sport in the twentieth and twenty-first centuries

By the beginning of the twentieth century, sport had evolved in line with the urbanised and industrialised society. It was governed by national governing bodies, which wrote the rules and oversaw competitions. The influence of NGBs spread far and wide across the globe and international competition began. The commercial side of sport was evolving, with professional performers and 'spectatorism' creating commercial clubs and purpose-built stadiums.

The working classes generally had Saturday afternoons off, which consequently became the time for sport. Church and factory teams sprang up and many entrepreneurs with an eye for making money also set up teams. These teams required regular fixtures, and clubs began to pay players to attract spectators and better players. The more spectators they attracted, the more money there was to pay players. In 1888, an elite group of professional teams from the Midlands and North came together to form the Football League. Cricket's County Championship similarly developed into a system of regular fixtures with points and a champion.

In rational sport, few played and many watched. This contrasts with the popular recreation of the seventeenth and eighteenth centuries, when many played and few watched.

Globalisation

Sport is now played all over the world. The sports that were developed in the UK at the end of the nineteenth century have spread around the world and many countries now play football, cricket and rugby — although some sports have their own distinctive styles in different locations. For example, Australian Rules and American football are both based on rugby.

With the rise of quicker travel, especially by air, and the media's move to satellite and broadband broadcasting, sports competitions have become global events. The Olympic Games now boasts a television audience of over 4 billion.

Media corporations are willing to pay large amounts of money to secure the exclusive rights to screen events. The huge audiences also make the events attractive to sponsors, who can pay to have their logos and brands seen around the stadiums and on the players' clothing. This 'shop window' created by the globalisation of sport is used by countries, groups and individuals for political and propaganda purposes.

Between 1960 and 1990, the USA and the USSR spent huge amounts of money trying to outdo each other in sport. A win at the Olympics was seen as proof that one political system was better than the other. Each country also boycotted an Olympics and used its power and influence to persuade other countries not to take part. This seriously affected the Olympic Games of 1980 and 1984.

Americanisation and commercialism

Sport is now big business. Sporting bodies increasingly turn to the private sector for financial support. This system of funding through sponsorship and fees from the media first developed in American sport. It has now crossed the Atlantic and is referred to as 'Americanisation'.

There is a direct link between the funding of sport and the media. Media coverage brings sponsors and advertising to sport, which are now essential for a sport to remain viable. Companies sponsor sports mainly as a means of cheap advertising — a way of getting into the public's living room. This is referred to as sport's 'golden triangle'.

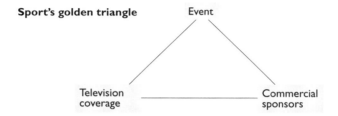

Sport's golden triangle

Event

Television coverage

Commercial sponsors

The move towards private funding has changed the main ethic in sport from the traditional 'playing for the love of the game' to a more commercial 'win at all costs' attitude. This has brought a move towards an 'open' focus where performers are free to earn money from sport.

What the examiners will expect you to be able to do

- Explain the term globalisation with reference to sport.
- Explain the influence that the 1984 Olympics had on future global games.
- Describe the rise of spectatorism and explain its influence on sport in the twentieth century.
- Comment on the development of commercialisation and Americanisation in UK sport.

Tip Make sure you can identify examples of Americanisation and the influence of commercialism on other global sports events.

Deviance in sport

All sports have rules and deviance occurs when participants break these rules. This **cheating** is an important issue in modern sport.

Cheating is not a new concept — we know that the ancient Olympians took tonics to try to improve their performances. Some people would argue that cheating is an important element in sport and that without it sport would be dull.

Sport has many written rules but there are also unwritten ones, and these make investigation of deviance more complicated.

Sportsmanship and gamesmanship

The Olympic ideal is based around the philosophy of **sportsmanship** — people conforming to the written and unwritten rules of sport. The idea of **fair play** means that you treat your opponents as equals and, although you want to beat them, you will do so only by adhering to the rules and a code of conduct that has been developed in the sport through tradition.

The alternative dynamic in sport is known as **gamesmanship** — where you use whatever means you can to overcome your opponent. The only aim here is to win, and for most people it is not a question of breaking the rules, but more bending them to their advantage.

Performance-enhancing drugs

Drug abuse has been one of the main areas of deviance in sport over the last few years. It is not clear whether the actual level of drug taking has increased or whether we are now more aware of it because testing systems have improved.

Most performance-enhancing drugs originated as genuine medical treatments but athletes have used the side effects to improve their athletic performance. The range and availability of these types of drugs is increasing, making control difficult.

Performance-enhancing drugs commonly used in sport include:
- **anabolic steroids** such as Nandrolone — these help to build muscle and aid faster recovery from training
- **peptide hormones** such as EPO — EPO increases the number of red blood cells in the body and therefore raises the oxygen-carrying capacity, which has a beneficial effect on aerobic activity
- **human growth hormone** such as somatotrophin — this increases the number of red blood cells, boosts heart function and makes more energy available by stimulating the breakdown of fat
- **stimulants** such as amphetamines — these raise the heart rate and reduce feelings of fatigue
- **diuretics** — help the body to lose fluids, which is useful in sports where athletes need to maintain a certain weight, e.g. boxing and horse racing

Taking performance-enhancing drugs to improve performance and increase the chances of winning is a good example of gamesmanship. The rewards of winning have tempted many athletes to cheat, particularly in one of the most prestigious athletics events — the 100 metres sprint. Starting with Ben Johnson in 1988, several of the world's top sprinters, including Linford Christie, Tim Montgomery and more recently Dwain Chambers, have tested positive and received bans for taking performance-enhancing drugs.

Media attention has focused mainly on the use of steroids. These are artificial male hormones that allow performers to train harder and for longer. In the past they have been difficult to trace because they are not taken immediately before performance. Athletes take them during the preparation phase, usually in the 'closed' season. The decision to start testing athletes at any time in the year has led to a breakthrough in detection.

There is a fine line between what is classed as a legal supplement and what is classed as an illegal drug. Some athletes have tested positive although they claim to have taken only cough mixture or other over-the-counter products. A substance is illegal only if it is on the IOC Medical Commission's list of banned substances. Athletes with access to highly qualified chemists and physiologists may be able to keep one step ahead by taking substances that have not yet been banned.

WADA and the fight against drugs

The World Anti-Doping Agency was established in 1999 and charged with promoting and coordinating the fight against doping in sport. WADA is governed by a board that includes representatives from the major international sporting organisations, including the IOC, as well as sports ministers from a number of governments. So far, its primary aim has been to fund a considerable increase in the annual number of drug tests and to produce a world anti-doping code. The main focus of this code is to regain athletes' confidence in doping control policy and to develop a framework that is consistent in its application, effective in its management and which respects and promotes the rights of athletes.

Future developments in deviance

Genetic engineering is a major new threat to the integrity of international sport, and one of WADA's main concerns. It could be used to fine-tune drugs to suit an athlete's genetic composition, and the drugs will be untraceable. A more sinister approach would be to use the technology to modify the cells of newly fertilised eggs to produce 'super' athletes.

What the examiners will expect you to be able to do

- Understand the concepts of sportsmanship and gamesmanship.
- Understand the reasons why performers take performance-enhancing drugs.
- Understand the role that WADA plays in attempting to reduce deviance in international sport.
- Discuss the future of deviance in sport.

Performance pathways

Key points

- The **sporting pyramid and its levels** — foundation, participation, competition, elite.
- The roles of key UK agencies including **UK Sport**, **Sport England**, **Sport Scotland**, the **Welsh and Northern Ireland Sport Councils**, **Youth Sport Trust**.
- The traditional and contemporary **pathways** in sport.
- The process of **talent identification** and **talent development**.

Sporting pyramid

The different levels of sport can be represented best as a pyramid. Such a concept is used by many sports organisations to develop a continuum of participation from the foundation level to the elite level. In theory, the broader the base of participation, the greater is the elite pool from which a society can select. There is also a link from the elite level to the base: success in sport creates role models, who can inspire people at the bottom of the pyramid — especially younger people — to get involved in sport.

The sporting pyramid

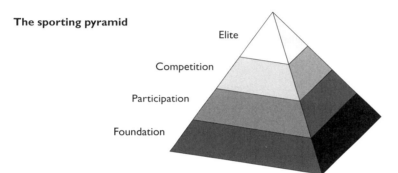

Tip It may be easier to revise if you use examples from the sport you play when referring to the different levels of the sporting pyramid.

There are four levels of performance within the pyramid:
- The **foundation level**, also known as the grass roots level, is mainly associated with young children being introduced to sport and learning the fundamental motor skills. In the UK, schemes such as TOP Sport and Dragon Sport have been used by the sports councils to promote participation at this level.
- At the **participation level**, older children are beginning to play full-scale sport, often for teams based in school or the community. The School Sports Coordinators programme and the Sports Education and Step into Sports initiatives are examples of strategies used to encourage participation at this level.
- The **competition level** is associated with participants who are committed to performing in formal, organised competition at higher club and regional level. Participants will usually train for their chosen sport and be members of a local sports club or organisation.
- The **elite level** is where elite athletes perform at a national and/or international level. For many of these performers, sport is their main focus or career. They receive funds either as professionals or through grants and awards from sports organisations such as the Sports Lottery Fund.

Role of key UK sports agencies
There are three key agencies that oversee sport in the UK today.
- **UK Sport** is responsible for the management of elite sport in the UK, e.g. the UK Sports Institute Network (UKSI), World Class Performance Programme.

- **Sport England** is responsible for advising, investing in and promoting community sport to create an active nation, e.g. promoting a sports tool kit, distributing money from the lottery sports fund (in the other home countries this role is undertaken by the respective Sports Council).
- The **Youth Sport Trust** has responsibility for all sport and activity that involves young people in and out of school, e.g. TOP programmes, specialist sports colleges and school sport partnerships, Physical Education, School Sport and Club Links (PESSCL) strategy.

Traditional and contemporary pathways

In the UK, there have been two traditional pathways for aspiring athletes and performers:
- education — school, regional teams, university, elite club
- club — local junior club, senior club, elite club

Which pathway a young person took was largely determined by the sport, although in sports such as rugby and netball, both approaches were available. Recently there has been a move towards the club structure, since the funding and support managed by UK Sport is available through governing bodies and clubs. The PESSCL strategy and role of the specialist sports colleges has gone some way to bringing the two pathways closer. Reflecting the traditional pathway in sport (school — club — international), 50% of British Olympic medal winners over the last 50 years have come from the private education sector (which constitutes only 7% of the total British population).

Game Plan

In December 2002, the UK government published Game Plan, a strategy for delivering the government's sport and physical activity objectives. Game Plan sets out two main aims:
- to initiate a major increase in participation in sport and physical activity, primarily because of the significant health benefits from being active and to reduce the growing costs of inactivity faced by the country (especially the alarming rise in obesity)
- to create a sustainable improvement in success in international competition, particularly in the sports that matter most to the public, primarily because of the national 'feel good factor' associated with winning

Game Plan sets the ambitious targets of:
- 70% of the population being reasonably active by 2020
- British and English teams and individuals sustaining rankings within the world's 'top five', particularly in more popular sports

Talent identification and development

Concept of talent identification

Talent identification (talent ID) is the process of identifying potential sporting talent in young people, and then providing supportive pathways that allow them to progress and fulfil this talent.

The identification of future sporting potential is not an easy task. Most of the current systems use physical characteristics and capacities that have been mapped against specific sports. However, achieving success in top-level sport also requires high levels of desire, determination and mental toughness, which are not so easy to measure and identify.

History of talent development in East Germany and Australia

East Germany is often credited with being one of the first nations to develop the concept of talent identification. A relatively small country, East Germany had a population of only 16 million but was one of the top four nations in international sport.

The success of East Germany's sports system was a direct result of its talent identification programme, which became an integral part of school sport at primary level. Every child was screened for sporting potential at the age of seven, and those who were successful were transferred to a sports boarding school where more time could be devoted to sports training. Those who continued to make progress graduated to a high-performance centre or sports institute. The athletes could now devote themselves full-time to preparation at one of eight national centres where they had access to top-class facilities, the best coaches and an array of sports science and technical support. This model has been adopted around the world.

In Australia, the AIS functions in a similar way to the East German high-performance centres. Born out of Australia's disappointing performance at the 1976 Olympics in Montreal, the Australian government undertook a review of its elite sports system. The outcome was a decision that the country needed a central focus for identifying and nurturing its sporting talent. The AIS offers scholarships to over 600 elite athletes in 32 different sports. It employs 75 full-time coaches and offers athletes top-class training facilities alongside sports science and medical back-up. A further seven satellite institutes are now based in Australia's state capitals.

Talent development in the UK

In 2000 the UK government produced its vision for sport for the forthcoming decade. A document entitled 'A sporting future for all' set out plans for talent identification and development in the UK.

Within the **National Framework for Sport**, a partnership between the UKSIs and the national governing bodies has been developed to facilitate the systematic identification of talent and fast-track development programmes in targeted sports towards London 2012.

UK Sport has proposed that it takes 6–8 years for a promising athlete to reach medal-winning potential. For the first time, dedicated talent ID specialists are employed around the country looking for potential talent. There is a specific focus on the new Olympic sports (basketball, handball and volleyball).

Other talent identification programmes include:
- Project Swap Shop
- Sports Search

- UK School Games
- Talented and Gifted Performance
- World Class Programme
- Talented Athlete Scholarship Scheme (TASS)
- Advanced Apprenticeship in Sporting Excellence (ASE)

What the examiners will expect you to be able to do

- Describe the different levels of the sporting pyramid.
- Explain the traditional pathways open to performers in the UK.
- Explain the role that key agencies play in managing the sporting pyramid.
- Describe and explain the concepts of talent identification and talent development.

Lifelong involvement

Key points

- The concept of **mass participation**, **lifetime sports** and the **constraints** on participation.
- The Sport for All campaign and other **reformative** policies.
- How the key sports agencies identify **target groups**.
- Technical developments and **cultural trends**.

Lifetime sports

Sport for All campaign

The Sport for All campaign was launched in 1972. It highlights the value of sport and promotes the idea that sport should be accessible to all members of the community. The campaign initially hoped to increase the opportunities for sport and recreation through developing more facilities, and by educating the public on what is available. More recently, the campaign has diversified to target groups of the community that remain under-represented in sport. Campaigns such as '50+ and All to Play For' (aimed at older people) and 'What's Your Sport?' (aimed at women) have followed.

Sport England has divided the 'market' for sports participation into four segments. For each segment there is a targeted strategy to reduce drop-out, increase participation, and improve attitudes towards physical activity.

- **Sporty types**
  Description: approximately 20% of the population. People who participate in sport and are keen to continue. These people will play almost regardless of government intervention.
  Sport England's action plan: safeguard provision of sporting opportunities and develop pathways to elite sport

- **Mild enthusiasts**
  Description: approximately 16% of the population. People who participate in sport but could do more. They know the benefits of sport and could be encouraged to do more.
  Sport England's action plan: increase access, reduce drop-out and foster enthusiasm
- **On the subs bench**
  Description: 44% of the population. People who do not currently participate but who could be persuaded to if it was made easy enough. These people may have little time or energy and feel they are not sporty enough.
  Sport England's action plan: remove barriers, offer incentives and take sport to them.
- **Couch potatoes**
  Description: 20% of the population. People who don't participate and don't want to. They have a negative attitude towards sport — often established at an early age. These people have little interest in sport/fitness and like to put their feet up.
  Sport England's action plan: raise awareness, promote the health benefits and change attitudes to physical activity at a young age.

The government and key sports agencies believe that participation in sport and physical activity can:
- help people to lead healthier lifestyles
- create safer communities
- promote positive behaviour and confidence
- improve educational attainment
- help to build social networks within communities
- reach out to and engage with disaffected people

Concept of mass participation
The basic premise of sport for all is that the opportunity to take part in sporting activity and physical recreation should be a basic human right. However, there are constraints that prevent many people from taking part. The aim of mass participation is to break down any constraints, and encourage as many people as possible to take up active lifestyles.

There are many benefits for society in promoting mass participation in sport. **Intrinsic** benefits of physical activity include:
- it promotes mental and physical health
- it is a positive use of spare time
- it is an important emotional release

Extrinsic benefits are that:
- people will be fitter and healthier, so there will be less strain on the health system
- crime and antisocial behaviour may be reduced if people are engaged in physical activity
- there may be economic benefits from increased numbers taking up an active lifestyle
- this may be attractive to investors and companies looking to relocate

Constraints on mass participation

The basic requirements for an active lifestyle include:
- a basic level of **physical fitness**
- the skills required to play sport (**ability**)
- access to kit and equipment (**resources**)
- **leisure time** away from the demands of work and other duties

Lifestyles have changed over the last century — the development of transport and other technological advances have meant a move towards a more sedentary lifestyle. Work and leisure often require much less physical activity than they used to. There are now concerns about the lack of fitness among young people and the rise of diseases such as obesity and cardiac problems.

Cultural factors

Many people do not have equal access to sport, often as a result of discrimination due to cultural variables. A number of so-called **target groups** can be identified. These are groups that find it difficult to access sport and recreation.

There are five main cultural factors that can lead to discrimination in sport:
- gender
- social class/economic status
- ethnicity (race and religion)
- age
- ability/disability

Discrimination can be said to affect the following areas in sport:
- opportunity
- provision
- esteem

Opportunity

There may be barriers to an individual's participation in an activity. In the UK, most sport takes place in clubs run on a voluntary basis. These clubs are often elitist organisations. Clubs work on membership systems and membership is controlled either by the ability to pay fees or, in some cases such as golf clubs, election to club membership. This often limits membership to certain members of the community.

Another consideration for the individual is whether he/she has the time to play. Women in particular are frequently faced with this problem. The demands of work and family often mean that they have little leisure time, which accounts in part for the low levels of female participation in sport.

Provision

Are the facilities that allow participation available to you? Living in an inner-city area might discriminate against you because there is often little provision in these areas. Equipment is also required, which can be expensive. Those on low incomes may be discriminated against unless equipment is available free or can be hired cheaply.

Esteem

This is concerned with the views and judgements of society. In many cultures societal values dictate that women should not take an active part in sport, or if they do it should be confined to 'feminine' sports such as gymnastics and not 'macho' pursuits such as football and rugby. These judgements are based on the traditional roles that men and women have taken in society and may be difficult to break.

Stereotypes

Stereotypes may lead to myths in sport, leading to discrimination. Common sports myths are that 'black people can't swim' and that 'women will damage themselves internally if they do hurdles'. Myths are based on very little truth, but often become an important aspect in selection and opportunity.

Stereotypes and myths can become self-fulfilling prophecies. Even the people they discriminate against may believe they are valid and conform to the stereotype by displaying their appointed characteristics and choosing the sports that fit them.

Reformative policies

The strategies and initiatives put forward to encourage people into physical activity are called **reformative policies**. Some national policies have already been mentioned. Sport England's Active Places programme aims to give people access to an internet database of facilities and clubs in their local area. The PESSCL strategy developed by the Youth Sport Trust provides more opportunities for school-aged children to take part in physical activity, and encourages links between schools and clubs so that they will continue to play when they leave school.

At a local level, sports centres often use a system called programming, where time is provided for particular target groups. Examples include swimming sessions for women only, or for the over-50s. Another strategy is to offer concessions for particular groups of customers.

The work of key sports agencies

Agency	Role
Women's Sports Foundation	Encourages, promotes and celebrates active and healthy women and girls
Kick It Out	Football's anti-racism campaign; works at all levels of football to tackle racial abuse and encourage ethnic minority participation
English Federation of Disability Sport	National body responsible for developing sport for disabled people in England

Technical developments and cultural trends

There are a number of developments and trends that may affect people's decisions to take up sport and physical activity.

- There has been a huge growth in private gyms and health clubs: the issue here is the cost of membership.
- Fashion and the role of media: this can have a positive effect — there has been an upsurge in both ballroom dancing and ice-skating due to high-profile television shows featuring these two activities.
- Technology linked to access: equipment and sports kit is getting cheaper and of a better standard — again, this should have a positive effect.
- Adrenaline and adventure sports have witnessed a rise in popularity over the last decade, especially 'street sports' such as rollerblading and skateboarding: this has been facilitated by many local authorities building skate parks.
- The impact of the 2012 Olympic Games being awarded to London.

Long-term athlete development

Key points

- The long-term athlete development programme creates pathways to introduce people into sport.
- It also creates pathways that allow people to progress in sport.

LTAD programme

The concept of long-term athlete development (LTAD) is credited to an article written by elite sports consultant Istvan Balyi in 2002. It was adopted by UK Sport in 2006 as the model for elite sports development in the UK. The majority of NGBs in the UK have now produced an LTAD pathway for their sport.

Tip Check out your NGB website. Has an LTAD been produced for your sport?

The basic LTAD programme identifies four key stages:
- FUNdamentals
- Training to Train
- Training to Compete
- Training to Win
(Another stage is sometimes added: retirement.)

There are two models:
- **Early specialisation sports** require early specialisation in training, for example gymnastics, swimming, figure skating, diving and table tennis.
- **Late specialisation sports** require a generalised approach to early training, for example athletics, team sports, combat sports and rowing. It is suggested that specialist training for these types of sports should commence after the age of ten.

What the examiners will expect you to be able to do

- Explain the concepts of Sport for All and mass participation.
- Describe and apply Sport England's participation segments.
- Explain the constraints of participation and the term 'target group'.
- Discuss examples of reformative policy.

Tip Look for local examples of target group programmes and reformative policies at your local sports centre. Don't forget to use these in your examination answers.

Questions
&
Answers

This section contains questions similar in style to those you can expect to see in the Unit 1 examination. The limited number of example questions means that is impossible to cover all the topics and all the question styles, but they should give you a flavour of what to expect. The responses shown are real students' answers to the questions.

There are several ways of using this section:

- Hide the answers and try the questions yourself. It needn't be a memory test — use your notes to see whether you can make all the points you need to.
- Check your answers against the candidates' responses and make an estimate of the likely standard of your response to each question.
- Check your answers against the examiner's comments to see if you can appreciate where you might have lost marks.
- Check your answers against the terms used in the question — did you *explain* when you were asked to, or did you merely *describe*?

Examiner's comments

All candidate responses are followed by examiner's comments. These are preceded by the icon ⮱ and indicate where credit is due. In the weaker answers, they also point out areas for improvement, specific problems and common errors, such as lack of clarity, weak or non-existent development, irrelevance, misinterpretation of the question and mistaken meanings of terms.

Plyometric training

(a) Explain the concept of plyometric training and identify the type of athlete most likely to benefit from it. (4 marks)

(b) Describe a plyometric exercise suitable for an athlete of your choice and identify any potential risks associated with this type of training. (4 marks)

Total: 8 marks

■ ■ ■

(a) There is 1 mark for identifying the correct type of athlete. Any power athlete or athlete requiring muscular strength, power and coordination would be a suitable answer.

There are 3 marks for three of the following concepts:
- muscles perform a significant eccentric contraction/are forcibly pre-stretched
- provides the potential for a greater concentric contraction, which produces a greater stress and therefore a greater potential for adaptation
- can be made sport-specific
- recruitment of type IIa and IIb fibres

(b) There is 1 mark for the plyometric exercise chosen, provided it is suitable for the named athlete. There is a maximum of 2 marks available for the description of the exercise and a maximum of 3 marks for the associated risks. For example, for a hockey player:
- bounding and two-footed jumps
- jumping high and landing low with full bend in the knees

The risks include:
- greater load placed on the muscle during the eccentric contraction
- high susceptibility to DOMS
- high susceptibility to joint/soft tissue injury
- not suitable for young athletes before physical maturity
- lack of variance/boredom

■ ■ ■

Candidates' answers to Question 1

Candidate A

(a) Plyometric training involves bounding or jumping continuously for a short time and then sprinting for a short time. The basic rule is a concentric contraction quickly followed by an eccentric contraction with the aim of improving explosive power. The idea is that the muscles are worked intensively to the point of exhaustion. Consequently they are vulnerable and could not act to protect oneself in an emergency. Because of this, they repair themselves, becoming bigger and stronger so that next time they will be better able to cope with the same intense exercise.

Athletes who benefit from this type of training include 100 m sprinters, because it develops both muscle strength and the power of muscular contractions so that the athletes can compete more effectively in their explosive sport.

> This wordy answer scores 1 mark only — for identifying that a **100 m** sprinter would benefit from plyometric training. The explanation of plyometrics scores no marks because the types of contraction are in the wrong order.

Candidate B

(a) • A high jumper would perform plyometrics.
- It produces a greater stress to the muscle and so encourages a greater improvement.
- An example of plyometrics is jumping off a gymnastics box.
- On landing, the muscles perform a powerful eccentric contraction.
- This enables the high jumper to perform a bigger concentric contraction on jumping again immediately after landing.

> The candidate uses the example of a high jumper to illustrate understanding of the training. Writing a separate sentence for each point rather than a continuous paragraph is an acceptable way of answering this type of question. Candidate B scores all 4 marks.

Candidate A

(b) For a 100 m sprinter, plyometric training involving bounding for 20 m, followed by a short sprint of 50 m, would be suitable. This should be done at a high intensity. Plyometric training does carry some potential risks. If the athlete is not fully warmed up, bounding — which should be done as intensively and maximally as possible — carries the risks of muscle strain or hamstring tear.

> This brief description of the exercise (i.e. bounding) scores 1 mark, as does the description of the potential risks. Candidate A scores 2 marks.

Candidate B

(b) High jumper, performing depth jumps.

The athlete starts from the top of a bench and jumps down. During the landing the muscle groups are working eccentrically and come under extreme force. The athlete then immediately takes off and jumps up, performing a concentric muscle contraction.

The distance reached on the spring could be measured and the athlete could try to improve on that. Alternatively, the athlete could jump over a pole laid horizontally, the height of which is increased over time.

The training could be dangerous and could result in tearing or damaging the quadriceps muscle or the soft tissue in the knee.

> Candidate B names and describes the exercise well and identifies the associated potential risks. This is a good answer, scoring all 4 marks.

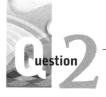

Muscle fibre types and sports activities

(a) The different types of muscle fibre are sometimes called type I, type IIa and type IIb. Give the alternative name for each type of fibre and identify a sport suited to each one. (3 marks)

(b) Identify suitable methods of training to develop each fibre and describe the adaptations that should occur. (9 marks)

Total: 12 marks

■ ■ ■

(a) The alternative name for type I fibres is slow twitch. Any predominantly aerobic-dependent sport would be a suitable answer.

Type IIa fibres are also called fast-twitch-oxidative-glycolytic fibres (FOG). Suitable sports are speed-endurance events, e.g. 400 m and 800 m on the track and 200 m in the pool.

Type IIb fibres are called fast-twitch-glycolytic fibres (FTG). Suitable sports are power/anaerobic events, e.g. 100 m sprint and shot put.

(b) For each type of muscle fibre, there is a maximum of 3 marks from the marking points given below.

For type I (slow twitch) fibres, continuous, fartlek or interval training would be suitable. The adaptations that should occur include:
- increased myoglobin
- increased density of mitochondria
- increased glycogen stores in muscle
- capillarisation in muscles
- a greater percentage of type I fibres, as a result of type IIa fibres developing slow-twitch characteristics
- being more efficient in aerobic conditions

For type IIa (FOG) fibres, interval, speed, circuit, weight and fartlek training would all be suitable. The adaptations that should occur include:
- increased myoglobin
- increased density of mitochondria
- increased glycogen stores in muscle
- increased tolerance of lactic acid
- capillarisation in muscles
- being more efficient in speed-endurance conditions
- a greater percentage of type IIa fibres, as a result of type IIb fibres developing type IIa characteristics

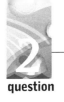

For type IIb (FTG) fibres, interval, speed, weight and circuit training would be suitable. The adaptations that should occur include:

- increased stores of PC (phosphocreatine)
- increased tolerance of lactic acid
- larger muscle bulk
- a greater percentage of type IIb fibres, as a result of type IIa fibres developing type IIb characteristics
- being more efficient in anaerobic conditions

■ ▧ ■

Candidates' answers to Question 2

Candidate A

(a) Type I fibres are more commonly known as slow-twitch muscle fibres. This type of muscle fibre is suited to a long-distance runner because of its resistance to fatigue and ability to work aerobically for a long time.

Type IIa fibres are also known as fast-twitch-oxidative-glycolytic fibres. They are suited to middle-distance runners because of the balance of power and resistance to fatigue.

Type IIb fibres are also known as fast-twitch-glycolytic fibres. They are suited to sprinters because of their powerful contraction and large muscle diameter.

🖉 This is an excellent answer that warrants the full 3 marks. The candidate demonstrates understanding of this area by justifying the choice of sport. The question does not ask for this, but if time permits it can be a useful ploy. In some cases, it might enable an examiner to award a mark that may have been in doubt because of a confused description.

Candidate B

Type I: slow twitch, marathon runners
Type IIa: FOG, 800 m runners
Type IIb: FTG (fast-twitch fibres), 100 m sprinters

🖉 Candidate B has provided the absolute minimum required. However, the question has been answered correctly, so the candidate scores 3 marks. This type of answer can save time. However, it runs the risk of perhaps being too brief and so, on occasion, missing marks.

■ ▧ ■

Candidate A

(b) Weight-training would be a suitable method to use to improve type I muscle fibres. Type I muscle fibres have a low force and speed of contraction. Weight-training will increase the force of contraction and muscle diameter, allowing athletes to have all the aerobic qualities these fibres contain and to have powerful contractions so that they can run, cycle or swim faster.

For type IIa fibres, interval training can be used. This will increase muscle diameter and hopefully, therefore, increase energy stores in the muscle.

Type IIb fibres have great explosive power but can only work maximally for a short time. They are easily fatigued. To develop these muscle fibres, interval training can be used to increase resistance to fatigue and lactic acid build-up.

✍ Although weight-training can be used for slow-twitch fibres, it is not the most usual method and so to gain a mark Candidate A would need to state that the training would be with a light weight and performed for many repetitions. For type IIa and IIb fibres, Candidate A's answer is too brief for the full mark allocation, but it gains 2 marks in each case, giving a total of 4 marks out of 9.

Candidate B

(b) Slow-twitch fibres: continuous training will produce an increase in capillarisation and increased aerobic capacity.

Fast-twitch FOG fibres: circuit training will encourage further capillarisation in the muscles. Type IIb and type I fibres will begin to adopt type IIa characteristics.

Fast-twitch FTG fibres: weight-training will increase anaerobic capacity, brought about by an increased size of fibres, which means that they will be able to hold larger stores of PC and ATP.

✍ This is a competent, detailed answer, which is split into three sections. In each section, the candidate identifies the method of training and then refers to the adaptations that are likely to occur. Candidate B scores all 9 marks.

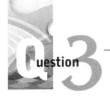

Effects of over-training

Training too hard with insufficient rest leads to deterioration in performance. Describe the symptoms likely to be experienced by an athlete who has trained too hard. (6 marks)

■ ■ ■

Any six from the following marking points would score 1 mark each:
- lethargy
- prone to injury or illness
- drop-off in performance
- loss of appetite
- moody
- excessive muscle soreness
- lack of motivation
- weight loss
- reduction in muscle mass

■ ■ ■

Candidates' answers to Question 3

Candidate A

Over-training may lead to deterioration in performance. It is indicated by various symptoms, including rapid weight loss and prolonged lack of appetite. An athlete may experience muscle soreness and have a greater chance of picking up an injury. There may be a lack of motivation to train. All these symptoms are ways in which the body is trying to tell the athlete that he or she is training too much.

This is a good, succinct answer, which scores all 6 marks.

Candidate B

DOMS is delayed onset muscular soreness. The symptoms are lack of flexibility and sore, tender muscles caused by acid or waste products. DOMS means a decreasing level of performance. It is caused by excessive eccentric contractions.

Candidate B has misunderstood the question and fails to score.

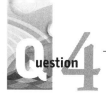

Flexibility training

Flexibility training is used to increase the range of motion at a joint. Name and describe two different types of flexibility training used to achieve this improvement.

(4 marks)

■ ■ ■

The types of flexibility training are:

- static — the muscle is taken to its limit and held under tension
- ballistic — momentum is used to force the fibres to stretch over a greater range
- PNF — the muscle is stretched to its limit and then performs an isometric contraction while stretched; this is repeated after relaxing
- active static — the performer stretches the body part
- passive static — the performer allows a partner to move the limb to the point of stretch

Any two of the above would earn 2 marks each.

■ ■ ■

Candidates' answers to Question 4

Candidate A

PNF can be used as flexibility training. This involves contracting the muscle before stretching it. This method is used to relax the muscle and allow it to be stretched slightly further each time the stretch is performed.

This is not a particularly well-answered question. The candidate has identified a single method of training when the question clearly asks for different *types*. The description of PNF is vague and confused. Candidate A scores 1 of the available 4 marks.

Candidate B

- PNF — taking a muscle to its stretched limit, performing an isometric contraction when at this point — stretch, contract, relax.
- Dynamic stretching — taking the joint and muscles through the range of movement likely to be experienced when performing.
- Static stretching — taking a muscle to its limit and holding.
- Ballistic — using momentum to force a muscle beyond its normal range of movement.

This is a detailed answer, which scores maximum marks. However, the candidate has ignored the question and wasted time by providing all four modes.

Fitness components

Identify and define two components of fitness required by a particular athlete, explaining the role of each component for that athlete. (6 marks)

■ ■ ■

There is 1 mark for each component of fitness identified, 1 mark for each correct definition and 1 mark for each explanation. For example, for a high jumper, any two of the following would gain 6 marks:

- Agility — the ability to change direction at speed while retaining control. The high jumper must change direction on take-off and also on going over the bar.
- Flexibility — the ability to move a joint through its complete range of motion. As the high jumper goes over the bar, the back must hyperextend.
- Power — strength × speed. On take-off the athlete must exert a maximal force as quickly as possible.

■ ■ ■

Candidates' answers to Question 5

Candidate A

Power (strength × speed) is a component of fitness required by a 100 m sprinter. It is needed for exploding out of the blocks at the start of a race. Speed is needed for sprinting to the finish line and hopefully winning the race. A 100 m sprinter may also need fast reaction times so that when the starting gun is fired, he or she is ready to push out of the blocks as quickly as possible to gain an advantage over the other athletes.

This single paragraph means that the examiner has to search to allocate the 5 marks scored. A better layout (for full marks) would have been:

- For a 100 m sprinter, power is required.
- It is defined as strength × speed.
- Sprinters need power so that they can explode out of the blocks at the start of a race.
- A 100 m sprinter may also need fast reaction times.
- This is the time taken from experiencing a stimulus to responding and reacting.
- Sprinters need quick reactions so that when the starting gun is fired, they are ready to push out of the blocks as quickly as possible to gain an advantage over the other athletes.

This answer would have scored the full 6 marks. It would also have been clear to the candidate that 6 marks were possible because six points were made.

Candidate B

Javelin thrower

Speed is the ability to put the body or body parts into motion quickly. The run up to the eventual throw needs momentum.

Explosive/maximal strength is the maximal force that can be exerted once only. The throw needs to be the maximum the athlete can produce.

Although it scores quite well (5 marks), this answer is too brief to be awarded the full 6 marks. The answer falls down on the reasons why the athlete requires the components of fitness.

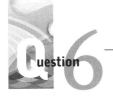

Fitness testing

Name a type of athlete and identify two components of fitness important for that athlete. Name one fitness test for each component and provide a brief description of the protocol for each test. (8 marks)

■ ■ ■

For example, a high jumper needs both flexibility and power.

A suitable test for flexibility is sit and reach:

- Sit with both legs outstretched and the soles of the feet flat against a vertical object.
- Reach forwards with both hands, keeping the legs straight and together.
- Measure the distance that can be reached either from or past the feet.

A suitable test for power is the standing sergeant jump:

- Stand with both feet together and measure the maximum reach height.
- From a standing position, jump as high as possible and measure the height reached.
- The difference between the two heights is proportional to the power generated.

1 mark is awarded for each component, 1 mark for each appropriate test and a maximum of 2 marks for each protocol description.

■ ■ ■

Candidates' answers to Question 6

Candidate A

For a 100 m sprinter, reaction time is an important component of fitness. A fitness test for this is the ruler drop. This involves somebody dropping a ruler from a certain height and the subject reacting as quickly as possible and catching it. The length of ruler that passes before the subject can catch it is recorded. Before the test begins, parameters must be set so that the test is clear: for example, where the ruler is dropped from, how many fingers the subject can use, whether the drop can be seen and so on.

This test is not really valid because it is not sport specific. The reliability of this test can be good, provided the parameters set are recorded and the test is carried out in the same way each time, with no external factors, such as wind.

Another component of fitness that a 100 m sprinter should have is speed. The 30 m sprint test could be used to test this component. Two cones are set 30 m apart and there are acceleration and deceleration areas before and after the cones. The athlete should pass the first cone at maximal speed, so a running start is required. The athlete sprints the 30 m without acceleration and the time is recorded. The test can be repeated three or four times and an average time calculated.

This test is valid for sprinters because it involves the same exercise as they do in their event — running.

Provided the track and the weather conditions are the same (or very similar) each time the test is performed, it is a reliable test.

🖉 This answer scores the full 8 marks. Indeed, it could have scored many more had the question asked for the application of the principles of validity and reliability to the tests. However, the question does not ask for that, so these parts of the answer cannot be credited. Candidate A has wasted time by providing this extra information.

Candidate B

Shot-putter

Maximal strength — 1 rep max test — tests the maximal strength exerted by the performer in one go.

Speed — 30 m sprint test. Two cones separated by 30 m, acceleration and deceleration points. Allowed acceleration beforehand.

🖉 This candidate scores 5 of the available 8 marks. Two components of fitness are identified, as is a test for each. However, the candidate offers no description of the protocol for the first test and only a very brief one for the second test.

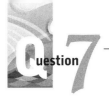

Question 7

Muscular–skeletal adaptations to aerobic training

Identify the adaptations to the muscular–skeletal system of an athlete that are likely to occur as a result of prolonged aerobic training. (5 marks)

■ ■ ■

There are 5 marks for any five of the following:
Muscular adaptations:
- increase in type I characteristics
- increase in myoglobin content
- increase in mitochondrial size/density
- increase in enzyme efficiency
- increase in localised muscular endurance
- decrease in subcutaneous fat levels

Skeletal adaptations:
- laying down of new stress lines/increase in bone density
- increase in ligament strength/elasticity
- increase in tendon strength/elasticity
- increase in production of synovial fluid
- increased thickness of articular cartilage

■ ■ ■

Candidates' answers to Question 7

Candidate A

There are many likely adaptations to the muscular–skeletal systems of an athlete as a result of prolonged aerobic training. You would expect the number of capillaries in the muscles to increase so that more blood, and therefore more oxygen, can get into the muscles while they are working, supplying more energy and allowing the muscles to continue working for longer. Cardiac output during exercise would increase. This is because, as a result of aerobic exercise, the heart would become bigger and stronger and, therefore, able to pump out more blood per beat. This would allow it to supply more oxygen to working muscles, more efficiently. This would mean better performance for the athlete. Stroke volume at rest and during exercise would also increase because of a bigger and stronger heart that has the capability to pump more blood and also has greater venous return efficiency. The increase in stroke volume would allow more oxygen to get to muscles and help increase cardiac output.

This is a poorly answered question, which is let down on many counts. First, it is wordy. This makes it difficult for the candidate to check that the five required points have been made. Second, it begins with an irrelevant sentence. Third, the candidate does what many others have done in the past when faced with similar questions — namely, making reference to cardiac or circulatory adaptations rather than sticking to muscular–skeletal ones. The question does not ask for an explanation of the benefit of these adaptations to future performance. Thus, the candidate scores 1 mark only, for stating that the number of capillaries in the muscles would increase.

Candidate B

- There is an increase in the myoglobin content of the muscle.
- There is an increase in capillarisation in the muscle.
- There is an increase in oxygen efficiency as more fibres begin to take on the characteristics of the slow-twitch muscle.
- Tendons increase in strength and elasticity.
- Cartilage is at risk of damage; there is wear and tear to hyaline cartilage.
- Bones might become stronger due to an increase in density.
- Bones are at risk of stress fracture.
- Ligaments increase in strength and show a slight increase in elasticity.

The candidate has listed eight anatomical adaptations to the two systems, which, time permitting, is a good idea. This could compensate for any point that may have inadvertently been repeated or answered in vague terms. The candidate scores comfortably the 5 marks available.

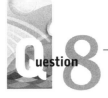

Fartlek training

Describe the main characteristics of fartlek training and explain its suitability for games activities. (4 marks)

■ ■ ■

The marking points are:

- training intensity/terrain varies
- allows longer distances to be covered/durations to be endured
- adaptable and can be used to focus on different fitness requirements
- incorporates active rest
- reflects the demands of games activities

■ ■ ■

Candidates' answers to Question 8

Candidate A

Fartlek (speedplay) training is a type of training in which the athlete changes intensity throughout the duration of the exercise. This allows the athlete to train for long periods of time, changing the intensity to use both the aerobic and anaerobic energy systems. It is suitable for games activities because it can be flexible in terms of fitness benefits. If carried out at varying low intensities, it can improve aerobic capacity. At higher intensities, resistance to lactate can improve. It can be specific to games players because they need differing types of fitness and during the games the intensity of exercise changes regularly, so the training prepares them well for this. A defender in football may only need to jog to maintain a good position or mark an opposing player when the team is attacking. However, when the team is defending, the player may have to sprint after the ball.

In its current format, this answer would score all 4 marks. However, it is unclear how much extra or unnecessary content has been included. Below is the same content with a better structure, making a clearer answer.

- Fartlek (speedplay) training is a type of training in which the intensity changes throughout the duration of the exercise.
- This allows the athlete to train for long periods of time, changing the intensity to use both the aerobic and anaerobic energy systems.
- It is suitable for games activities because it can be flexible in terms of fitness benefits.
- If carried out at varying low intensities, it can improve aerobic capacity. At higher intensities, it can improve resistance to lactate
- All these factors may be required by a games player.

Candidate B

Fartlek training is training at varying intensities for differing periods of time.

It enables athletes to cope with the varying intensity required, e.g. in football, a defender will often just need to jog around in a match, changing position in relation to the other players. However, the player may have to sprint after the ball for a short time.

Games require different times of high-intensity and low-intensity activity. Fartlek training caters for both these requirements.

e Because of the way in which the answer has been set out, the examiner is quickly able to ascertain that only three points have been made, rather than the four points indicated by the 4-mark allocation. Fartlek training has been defined correctly and its relevance for a games player justified. However, the candidate has not expanded on the characteristics of fartlek training, as required by the question, and scores 3 marks.

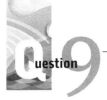

Combat sports in pre-industrial Britain

Discuss the importance of combat sports in Britain before 1800. Use examples to support your answer.   (5 marks)

■ ■ ■

✎ There are 4 marks available for four of the following points:
- preparedness for battle/war practice
- reflected hard, violent lifestyle/society
- entertaining/chance to gamble/wager
- part of education of nobleman/upper classes
- reinforced social status/etiquette/chivalric code
- lower classes compulsory/had to practise by law
- survival/hunting skills

There is a maximum of 2 marks for examples, e.g. jousting, archery, fencing, quarter staff, tournament.

■ ■ ■

Candidates' answers to Question 9

Candidate A

Before Britain underwent industrialisation, combat sports were considered the only real activity and essential sport. Before the 1800s there were many wars and invasions affecting Britain. The country saw that in order to maintain a strong defence, it was vital for the masses to practise and become experts in combat — they would be prepared for any event.

Two main types of combat sport were practised. One was jousting which provided military training for the upper classes. The other was archery, and it was compulsory for the lower classes to practise every Sunday after church. The main reason for this was because there was plenty of room for practice in the churchyard, and the trees from which the bows were made were also found there.

✎ This is a good answer that makes a number of points and backs them up with examples. However, it does not make enough points to score all the marks available. Candidate A scores 4 marks. Other points to make could include the need for self-defence skills and how combat was used to settle argument and feuds in the pre-industrial age.

Candidate B

Combat sports were important in Britain before 1800 as they kept the men fit for war and gave them the various skills needed in battle. It was compulsory to do sports such as archery; the King gave the order that every man had to practise. If people failed to do so, they would be punished.

The upper classes took part in combat sports to show the public how important and how high up they were in society. An example of this type of combat sport is jousting — you received points for attacking your opponents; the more hits you made, the more points you received. This sport also helped to develop horsemanship skills.

Archery is another example of a combat sport. It was compulsory for every man to own a bow. Archery practice and competitions would take place after church on Sundays. There would be many spectators and prizes for the best shots.

Candidate B gives good detail and makes enough points to score the 5 marks available.

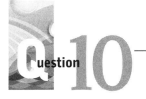

Sport in nineteenth-century public schools

Sport was an important element of life in nineteenth-century public schools. How were games used as a means of social control in public schools? (4 marks)

■ ■ ■

e There are 4 marks for four of the following points:
- keeping boys out of trouble/positive recreation
- catharsis/getting rid of aggression/frustration/excess energy
- means of settling scores/arguments
- educational values
- confined boys to school grounds
- fair play/sportsmanship ethos/developed discipline
- role of prefects/sixth-form controlling sports
- fitness/promotion of health

■ ■ ■

Candidates' answers to Question 10

Candidate A

The games practised, such as football, were useful as a means of social control because they aided in the development of personal sportsmanship and responsibility. Students were given the idea of enjoyment and the responsibility for learning as a team. Games were used to develop social skills that could be used later in life. Students passed on these sports to other areas in society. For instance, those students who went on to be priests or went to university passed on the rules. Sports in public schools were played throughout the British Empire and produced students with honourable characteristics, creating good soldiers for the army.

e This question focuses on the popular exam area of public school sport and its role in the historical development of sport in the UK. The candidate makes several valid points relating to character but misses the main point of sport being used as a means of channelling aggression and energy. Candidate A scores 2 marks.

Candidate B

Games were used a method of social control in public schools because it taught the boys how to work as a team. Games such as rugby, cricket and football were used as character-building methods of social control. In these games boys had to adhere to set rules and regulations, which helped develop discipline. Public schools were looking to produce leaders. The games required exercise and stamina, which would benefit the boys both in school, by allowing them to channel their energy, and in the wider society.

e Candidate B makes a range of points, including the key point about channelling aggression and energy, and names sports examples. Candidate B scores 4 marks.

Factors affecting participation

Sport for all is not yet a reality in the UK. How can a person's opportunity to participate in sport be affected by sociocultural factors? (5 marks)

■ ■ ■

Marks are awarded for five of the following:

- cost of taking part or low income
- lack of or cost of transport/limited public service
- ability, physique, stamina, fitness or level of disability
- social pressures, stereotypes or social constraints
- age — very old or young
- gender factors — females less likely to participate
- ethnic background, race or religion
- geographical factors — inner city/rural areas

■ ■ ■

Candidates' answers to Question 11

Candidate A

- Age — as you get older, it is harder to get to facilities because of the cost of transport, for example.
- Gender — women find it more difficult to access sports because of problems related to time and money.
- Race and religion — these may restrict a person from taking part in sport or recreation, e.g. Muslim girls may not be able to take part in sports such as swimming or gymnastics.
- Disability — some leisure centres cannot accommodate disabled people, e.g. they do not have ramps or disabled changing facilities.
- Economic status — people with less money cannot afford to participate in sport because in the UK we have to pay to play.

This answer makes at least five references to sociocultural factors and backs up each point with an explanation or examples. It scores the maximum 5 marks.

Candidate B

The age of the individual can affect his or her access to sport. The very young and the old find it more difficult to access sport and recreation. Where people live can also affect their access to sport. Those who live in rural areas may find it difficult to get to sports clubs. The ability of the individual can also be a factor, as can the fitness of the person. A person's gender is another factor — boys and girls play different sports.

This candidate attempts to identify five factors but fails to explain them fully or back them up with examples. In this type of question it is a good idea to put down one or two extra points if possible, to ensure that you score maximum marks. Candidate B scores 1 mark.

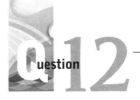

Amateurism at the Olympics

In 1896 the modern Olympic Games were established around the principle of the 'amateur ideal'. Discuss whether this principle is still relevant to Olympic performers in the twenty-first century. (12 marks)

■ ■ ■

The marking points are:

- de Coubertin's strong views on amateurism
- a copy of the English public school system
- elite class/social background of early Olympians meant that money was not an issue
- need for athletes to be able to pay their own way/no funding available from media or commercial sponsorship
- de Coubertin chose well-established amateur sports to make up the Olympic programme/ignored professional sports; professional sports were in the minority at the turn of the twentieth century
- upper-class bias through early games
- increase in nations and athletes from different cultural backgrounds began to dilute this influence as twentieth century developed
- this transition reflected the change in society and the growth of professional sports outside the Olympics
- 1980s saw the rise in the commercial nature of the games; performers becoming stars; sponsors increasingly interested in sport
- state manipulation of the concept of sponsorship; state-sponsored amateurs in USSR and college amateurs in USA
- sponsors and television now have biggest influence on the Games
- USA basketball dream team in 1992 broke the taboo of professional athletes in the Games
- games are now open but the majority of performers remain amateur or rely on state/lottery funding
- higher levels of performance has meant a need for full-time athletes

Counter-arguments could include:

- the majority of athletes remain 'amateur'
- media tend to focus on the elite or household names
- for many the Olympic ideal is simply getting to the Games

■ ■ ■

Candidates' answers to Question 12

Candidate A

Many of the principles around which the modern Olympic Games were established are still relevant in the twenty-first century. However, as time has passed, many changes in the structure and issues within society have taken place and these are reflected in the Olympic Games of the twenty-first century. The principle of the amateur ideal primarily means the love of sport and although many modern athletes may still feel this, there are many influences that now go against de Coubertin's established 'amateur ideal' and 'Olympic Dream'. In this essay, I will outline the meaning of the amateur ideal and discuss the similarities as well as the differences that exist in relation to this view in the twenty-first century.

The modern Olympic Games, established by Baron de Coubertin, were very much a celebration of sport. Competitors took part because of their love and enjoyment of their sport. The amateur ideal prevailed in that competitors did not receive any extrinsic rewards for their performances. Those who played for money or other extrinsic rewards were banned from competition at the Olympics. De Coubertin wished for the games to allow equal opportunity for everyone. He wanted the qualities he recognised and admired in the British public schools to be reflected in the attitude of competitors at the Games. He wanted every athlete to abide by the rules and acknowledge the concept of fair play. Perhaps most significantly, he stressed that the Olympic Games would not be an opportunity for political control. All these ideals were, of course, impossible due to the changes that were to occur socially, financially and politically during the twentieth century.

The Olympic Games of the twenty-first century now fully support the idea of professionalism. The amateur status of the modern Olympics rarely exists and competitors receive money from sponsors and grants from governments and sports organisations. This is accepted because of the time athletes now have to spend training and preparing. An Olympic athlete needs to train full time for most of the year and there is no possibility of being successful at the Olympics and continuing to have a job. Although the change from amateurism to professionalism has occurred, many athletes still compete for the love of their sport and not merely for the rewards that come with it.

Deviance in the Olympics is one of the aspects that counteracts de Coubertin's amateur ideal. For many athletes the success of a win has become more important than taking part. Therefore, in many respects, the concept of sportsmanship has now been replaced by gamesmanship. Many athletes will do anything to win, including tampering with equipment and taking banned performance-enhancing drugs.

The many changes that have taken place in the time from the re-emergence of the Olympic Games in 1896 to the Olympics of the twenty-first century go against the principles of the amateur ideal. However, the love of sport and desire to participate still exist along with those athletes who still practise good sportsmanship and show the honour that comes with competing for one's country.

✏ This answer broadly answers the question set. It starts with a good discussion about the concept of amateurism. What it lacks is any real depth or factual examples to back up the points made. The answer follows a sound structure and includes an introduction and a concluding paragraph. Candidate A scores 8 marks.

Candidate B

The modern Olympic Games still function around the amateur ideal; it is arguable that most of the athletes are 100% amateur. However, the boundaries are constantly being stretched through sponsorship and funding, along with the amount of media coverage the Olympics now enjoy.

The athletes who compete at the Games are not actually paid, but receive grants and scholarships from governments or lottery funds. These grants provide funding for the athletes to buy their own training equipment. They can also be used to provide adequate housing, food and supplies.

High-profile athletes may receive sponsorship deals from big brand names such as Adidas or Nike. These companies, as well as providing specialist equipment, tend to stretch the boundaries of what they provide for their athletes, and this brings into question whether the athletes are actually being given the same benefits as professionals. Some sponsors provide luxuries such as cars and other expensive gifts.

All this challenges whether the principle of the amateur ideal still exists. Another challenge to the amateur ideal is the increasing role that the media play in modern sport. Virtually all athletes who compete at the Games receive media coverage. This may mean that the athletes are used in advertising features in the same way as professional athletes. Moreover, the fact that they appear at the Games alongside professional performers raises the question whether they can be still labelled as amateur athletes. Stars such as Sir Steve Redgrave, Dame Kelly Holmes and Paula Radcliffe have been projected through the media frequently and no doubt have been able to secure huge sponsorship deals as a result of all the media coverage.

On the other hand, most athletes try to keep a low profile. Although they are at the elite level, they do not receive direct payment to compete and so the amateur ideal still exists. It is true to say that receiving sponsorship deals and supplements is not against the rules, and many athletes would do the same if put in a similar situation. The amateur ideal does still exist in the twenty-first century. Athletes go about their way of life in a professional, elite manner, but this is not reflected through any type of structured or one-off payments. The fact that many receive subsidies is just a reflection of current society. For most athletes these grants, which are still well below the average annual salary, mean that they can train and prepare for their events. Most of them will only get one attempt at the Olympics and will then have to return to a normal job and lifestyle.

✍ This response answers the question more directly and sticks to the point well. This essay is not as well structured and again lacks sufficient examples to back up the points made. However, it does discuss the issues well and raises a number of original thoughts. Candidate B scores 10 marks.